MW01289823

C. diff:
Our Gut-Wrenching
Road to Recovery

(A Learning and Healing Journal)

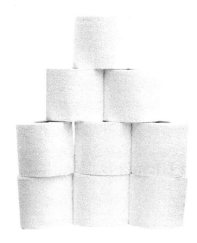

Ralph F. Voss
Glenda B. Weathers

(With a Foreword by Dr. Martin Rodriguez, M.D., Infectious Disease Medicine, University of Alabama at Birmingham)

C. DIFF: OUR GUT-WRENCHING ROAD TO

RECOVERY

(A Learning and Healing Journal)

by

Ralph F. Voss and Glenda B. Weathers

TABLE OF CONTENTS

Foreword

The discovery and development of antibiotic agents was one of the major and most significant scientific achievements of the 20th century. Antibiotics helped treat infections that were previously untreatable and dramatically improved the life expectancy of humans. The benefits provided by antibiotics are undeniable; however, now there are problems that have not been widely recognized as a result of using antibiotics. In recent years, doctors and scientists have found that bacteria are becoming more difficult to treat. In some cases, patients have died because there were no antibiotics available to treat an infection that had become resistant to all antibiotics. The Centers for Disease Control (CDC) and many other organizations and institutions are working to help educate physicians and the public about the appropriate use of antibiotics.

An emerging problem related to the use of antibiotics is infection by the bacteria *Clostridium difficile*. Decades ago, with the increasing use of antibiotics, physicians recognized that some patients developed diarrhea as a common side effect, likely caused by some changes in the gut bacteria triggered by the antibiotics. Most of these patients also had mild gastrointestinal distress that resolved once the antibiotics were discontinued. However, some patients who received antibiotics had moderate or severe diarrhea and abdominal pain, which in many cases led to hospitalization and sometimes to death. These patients who were severely ill were found to have extreme inflammation in the colon, and investigators found that some other antibiotics such as orally-given Vancomycin helped treat them. The cause for this problem was not identified until the 1970s, when *C. difficile* infection was found in these patients. Other research studies demonstrated that *C. difficile* is commonly found in hospitals, where patients are frequently exposed to this pathogen.

The normal human gut is usually resistant to symptomatic infection with this pathogen, likely because our normal gut bacteria keep it under check. However, after exposure to antibiotics for other infections in a hospital setting, many bacteria that normally live in our gut and provide health benefits are killed, leaving room for *C. difficile* to take over. This is the reason why *C. difficile* most often occurs after antibiotic use.

Eventually metronidazole, another antibiotic (usually marketed by the name Flagyl), was found to help with *C. difficile* colitis. Tests were developed to help diagnose *C. difficile* infection, and even though it was a common problem in hospitals and nursing homes, the general population was not very aware of its existence, so cases were mostly restricted to those locations. The number of cases therefore remained relatively stable for years. *C. difficile* infection, however, has more recently emerged as a major medical problem. The number of patients discharged from hospitals with a diagnosis of *C. difficile* infection doubled in the first decade of the 21st century, and studies have suggested that the mortality from this infection increased 10-fold. Recent estimates suggest that *C. difficile* contributes to more than 6000 deaths in the U.S. each year, and billions of dollars in excess healthcare costs. *C difficile* is more common in patients who are older than 65 and who have other medical problems, and it has become the 18th leading cause of death in this age group. Even though we now have antibiotics that help patients with *C. difficile* infection, killing the pathogen, some patients don't respond to these antibiotics and need more aggressive care, including surgery to remove the colon and other unconventional treatments. Clearly, the threat of *C. difficile* needs serious and closer scrutiny not only in the medical community but also in the general public.

The following story of contracting and battling *C. difficile* infection by Ralph Voss and Glenda Weathers shows just how dangerous the infection is, and serves a cautionary purpose for everyone.

Martin Rodriguez, M.D.

Associate Professor of Medicine

Division of Infectious Diseases

University of Alabama in Birmingham

Introduction:

What Is C. diff?

If you take antibiotics, especially what are called "broad spectrum" antibiotics, you can eventually be at risk for *Clostridium difficile*, "C. diff" for short. Broad spectrum antibiotics are what the name implies: they can kill a variety of bacteria that may be causing an infection, and therefore they are often prescribed, with healing results.[1] The potential problem is that a course of broad spectrum antibiotics can kill not only the bacterium causing the infection, but also other beneficial bacteria whose function is good for the normal operation of your intestines—what specialists call your "gut flora," a kind of ecology inside you that is in balance when you are healthy. If the antibiotics destroy too many beneficial bacteria and thereby disturb your intestinal ecology, sturdier, malevolent bacteria, such as C. diff, can flourish and make you sick—sometimes very sick,

---

1 There are many "broad spectrum" antibiotics, prescribed and marketed under various names, among them clindamycin, cephalixin, cefaclor, moxifoxacin, cetfazidim, imipenem, cephalosporins, flouroquinolones, and augmentin.

with recovery a difficult struggle.

C. diff is one of what are widely known as "super-bugs," medicine-resistant infectious strains that have proliferated in recent years. The term "super-bug," in fact, was first used in 1985. These super-bugs often linger in hospitals, nursing homes, and other areas where broad spectrum antibiotics are frequently used to treat frail, sick patients, though they are not limited to such areas. Regardless of wherever super-bugs are caught, they can be very difficult to get rid of, causing protracted and severe illness, even death. The origin of these super-bugs is generally believed by practitioners of medical science to be a result of a gradual evolution; that is, as various broad spectrum antibiotics have been increasingly prescribed by physicians for a wide variety of illnesses—even those caused by viruses, not bacteria— these medicines, once-considered "miracle drugs," have become less effective in knocking out bacteria-caused infections because these illness-causing bacteria have instead become stronger and more resistant to the antibiotics In other words, the strength and severity of the illness can grow while the antibiotics' ability to help the victim heal diminishes. In this way, "bugs" become "super-bugs," and the infections can grow worse, as happened to one of the authors of this book (Ralph) when he developed C. diff.

C. diff begins with mild stomach cramps and watery diarrhea three or four times a day, but in 70 to 80% of cases when C. diff is diagnosed, it can be cured after the first episode, ironically, with antibiotics—specifically, non-broad spectrum antibiotics such as Vancomycin (vancocin), Flagyl (metronidazole), or Dificid (fidaxomicin). However, sometimes the C. diff recurs once these specific antibiotics are discontinued, and in severe cases the specific antibiotics are largely ineffectual, making the infection far more threatening. In severe cases the stomach cramps become much more acute, and the watery diarrhea occurs more than ten times each day. Other symptoms can quickly escalate to include bloody stools, fever, nausea, and dangerous dehydration. If the severe infection persists, the patient's blood pressure drops, abdomen and legs swell, white blood cell count increases, and kidneys shut down. Muscle tissue begins to break down (rhabdomyolysis) and poison the bloodstream. Ulcerative colitis affects the colon, and surgery might even be necessary as the toxins damage the large intestine. Ralph suffered all these symptoms, but fortunately avoided colon surgery and recovered after having fecal transplants.

We hear you asking, "Fecal transplant? Really?" Yes, we know how that sounds. The treatment involves transplanting the stool of a gut-healthy person into the C. diff patient, and the transplanted healthy stool recolonizes the patient's gut with sufficient beneficial bacteria to restore the ecology of the patient's gut and heal the C. diff. In Ralph's case, the donor was his wife and co-author of this book, Glenda. Icky as it sounds, the fecal transplant worked where expensive non-broad spectrum specialty antibiotics including Vancomycin and Flagyl did not. We would have been willing to try the most expensive of all of these antibiotics—Dificid—if Ralph's illness had not become so protracted that we decided to aggressively pursue a fecal transplant instead, persuaded by what we'd heard about fecal transplant's effectiveness.

Our purpose in this book is to tell our story as a caution to readers who may routinely and unsuspectingly rely on broad spectrum antibiotics for minor illnesses that do not really require them for recovery, and to sound a caution to everyone that over-prescription of antibiotics in our culture today contributes to the rise of super-bugs like C. diff. Our book isn't meant to replace seeing a doctor, and it isn't a guide for self-diagnosis or self-reliant treatment; it is to suggest that rather than using fecal transplants as a *last* resort to bring healing relief to recurring C. diff sufferers, we think doctors should seriously consider using fecal transplants as an earlier option in treating these C. diff patients.[2]

---

2 The authors and publishers specifically disclaim any liability, loss, or risk, personal or otherwise, that is incurred as a direct or indirect consequence of the use and application of the contents of this book.

More about C. diff

To understand more about what C. diff is, we need to grasp some basics about the wide variety of bacteria that are important to our health. We commonly think that bacteria are bad because some of them can cause sickness. But some bacteria are also good for us, such as those present in yogurt and naturally-fermented sauerkraut, and the combinations of bacteria in our stomach and intestines help make our digestive system work properly. We need bacteria in our lives, but we need them to work *for* us and not *against* us. Although we did not know it at the time, Ralph's infection and subsequent recovery from C. diff happened to coincide with a growing interest among medical and scientific professionals in what researchers call the "normal human microbiome." This interest was reflected in a five year study, called the Human Microbiome Project, sponsored by the National Institutes of Health, published in 2008. The aim of the five year study was to catalog samples of bacteria from healthy volunteers in the United States in an attempt to understand the huge variety—and role—of microbes that live in and on our bodies. This huge variety, which numbers more than 10,000 microbial species and an estimated 100 trillion bacteria, almost always includes, even in healthy persons, some bad bacteria among the good. Yet, in healthy persons the good bacteria are sufficient in number and strength to control the bad pathogens that might otherwise cause illness, thus affecting our autoimmune systems. The University of Alabama in Birmingham (UAB) was among 80 institutions participating in the research that has provided a baseline database of microbes, the knowledge of which can provide a threshold for breakthroughs in effective treatments for a variety of illnesses.

Of particular interest here are the microbes that inhabit the gut; once the medical community more fully understands the relationship of good bacteria and bad, they can more effectively address such ailments as inflammatory bowel disease, including ulcerative colitis, Crohn's disease, and C. diff infection. In fact, when referring to the work of the Human Microbiome Project, UAB's Peter Mannon, M.D. (professor in the UAB School of

Medicine Division of Gastroenterology and Hepatology) indicates that the study's "reference database lays the foundation for advances in infectious, autoimmune and inflammatory diseases and potentially the identification of unique probiotics or even prescription fecal transplants to replace disease-causing microbiomes." (www.uab.edu/news/latest/item/2489-defined-healthy-microbiome-to-shake-up-understanding-of-many-diseases.) While "prescription" fecal transplants are not yet available as of this writing, they nonetheless show promise for the future, and certainly fecal transplants happened to play a significant role in what happened to us. As our story unfolds, we will tell you how fecal transplants (not the as-yet-to-be-developed-prescription-kind) saved Ralph from a terrible C. diff infection, and allowed both of us to resume our normal diarrhea-free lives. We spare no details because we think readers should not be squeamish about the stark realities that can come from severe C. diff infection.

How Does a Person Get C. Diff?

C. diff bacteria originate in fecal matter and therefore often exist on bed pans, toilets, bathing tubs, rectal thermometers and many other surfaces that are regularly touched by health care employees and their patients in hospitals and nursing homes. But they can actually be found anywhere fecal matter is or has been in even so much as a miniscule part of an environment. Because C. diff bacteria have an uncanny approach to survival, they are insidiously and sneakily dangerous. In fact, the active bacteria that have found their way onto the surfaces that we frequently touch—such as gas pump handles, currency, doorknobs, wall switches, television remote controls, back-of-seat airline trays, and the like—have very brief life spans, especially when eradicated with chlorine bleach. But all too often these bacteria can go into survival mode on those same surfaces by turning into spores and growing a shell that is resistant to most attempts to kill them. These spores can last for months on those familiar environmental surfaces where we are likely to touch them. When we fail to wash our hands frequently with soap and water, and accidentally ingest the spores by bringing our hands to our mouths, we introduce them into our digestive system.

Our guts, then, provide the spores with the rich environment they need for returning once again from spores to active C. diff bacteria. Even then, the C. diff bacteria might not cause serious problems *unless the person has recently taken a broad spectrum antibiotic.* Indeed, someone is more vulnerable to C. diff when antibiotics have been used to treat common infections. In attacking the bacteria that have caused the prior infection, the antibiotics also attack *all* the bacteria in the gut, disrupting the colony of microbes that keep us well and allowing the resistant C. diff bacteria to gain the upper hand. Severe diarrhea can be the result, leading to many of the serious problems mentioned above.

Treatment of C. diff

Of course, not all diarrhea is caused by C. diff. A person should therefore not assume automatically that a case of diarrhea is a case of C. diff. But certainly if diarrhea persists, even if loperamide (Immodium) is taken, a doctor should then be consulted. In most cases, the diarrhea caused by diagnosed C. diff can be successfully treated with Vancomycin (Vancocin) and/or metronidazole (Flagyl), antibiotics that have proved effective in 70 to 80 percent of cases. But in 20 to 30 percent of patients, the symptoms recur when Vancomycin or metronidazole treatment is discontinued. In severe cases, the antibiotics specifically aimed at C. diff, even fidaxomicin (Dificid), are often not enough and the diarrhea will persist unless and until a healthy community of bacteria is somehow restored in the gut. C. diff can be extremely stubborn, and in severe cases like Ralph's, the symptoms just keep recurring, making patients miserable, and in some cases even causing patients to die. We are not talking about a miniscule number of people; several sources report that annually half a million Americans experience C. diff infections, and of that half-million people, 14,000 die each year (See, for example, "Dire Infection, One-Day Cure," in the November, 2013 issue of *Good Housekeeping*, pp. 100-103). Hospitals and other health care facilities are acutely aware of the problems associated with C. diff. *The New England Journal of Medicine*, for example, reporting on a survey of health care-associated infections, indicates that "*Clostridium difficile* was the most commonly reported pathogen (causing 12.1% of health care-associated infections)."[3]

As mentioned above, C. diff is often treated with expensive antibiotics specifically targeted for C. diff: Vancomycin, an antibiotic administered orally but sometimes as an enema; Flagyl (metronidazole), another oral antibiotic; and another, currently even more expensive, oral drug named Dificid (fidaxomicin) that has proved effective in treatment. Obviously, for those who don't improve after using these special antibiotics,

---

3   March 27, 2014; pp. 1198-1208. PMID: 24670166. Found in
    Paper.medlive.cn, accessed January 10, 2015.

or have relapses, restoring the right community of bacteria in the colon is the key to recovery. Such restoration can sometimes be achieved by taking Vancomycin or Dificid along with probiotics. But such procedures too often prove disappointing. The Mayo Clinic website indicates that an *initial* onset of C. diff can be effectively treated in about 60% of cases using a tapered regimen of antibiotics; other sources estimate 70-80%. Yet, these same antibiotics prove less effective when treating recurrences of C. diff. Probiotics—certain bacteria that work to restore and maintain healthy bacterial balance—may also help, although they are more commonly used to help *prevent* digestive / elimination problems like C. diff, not to correct them; and anyway, by the time severe C. diff has set in, the digestive system often needs such a heavy and dramatic infusion of good bacteria that taking probiotics orally is generally insufficient to help effect recovery. Such an infusion can be supplied by fecal transplant—a "fecal microbiota transplant" in more technical terms—literally, taking stool from a healthy donor and placing it in the guts of the C. diff patient. Unpleasant as it sounds, such a fecal transplant is often a severe C. diff patient's best hope, for research indicates that this alternative therapy has a success rate greater than 90%.[4] However, many doctors and hospitals are unaware of the efficacy of fecal transplants, or they consider them experimental, or they (or their C. diff patients) consider them too "icky."

We didn't know any of this when Ralph got C. diff. Sure, he had taken antibiotics before, like most people, and had enjoyed the recovery such miraculous medicines seemed routinely to offer. And we had both heard of super-bugs before, but neither of us had ever heard of C. diff until Ralph got a bad case of it in late April, 2013, shortly after his 70th birthday. What follows is the story of the battle we both fought with C. diff. We are both super-bug survivors, and our purpose here is not to suggest that our pains and struggles are unique; on the contrary, we know that there are many others who contract and battle severe illnesses, many others who could tell stories of medical adversity every bit as painful, if not more so, than ours. We just want to share our

---

4   Mayo Clinic Website on clostridium difficile treatments, accessed January 8, 2015.

experience to inform and to caution readers about C. diff and to urge fecal transplant as a first-resort approach to healing patients suffering severe, recurring C. diff. Our inclusion of intimate details, which may at times seem excessive, is intended to convey, as honestly as possible, what it can mean to suffer and survive this horrific super-bug.

OUR STORY

*"Do not go gentle into that good night
Rage, rage against the dying of the light."*
Dylan Thomas

Little Did We Know

RALPH:

In 2009, shortly after I retired from a long teaching career,

I had gastric bypass surgery, chiefly for two reasons: first, and

typically for gastric bypass patients, I was obese, and persistent

efforts to lose weight via diet and exercise proved generally

ineffective; second, I was also an adult-onset (sometimes known

as "Type 2") diabetic, and research has shown that most obese

adult-onset diabetics who have gastric bypass surgery not only

lose weight but also experience the disappearance of diabetic

symptoms. In my case, both significant weight loss and cessation

of diabetic symptoms resulted from my gastric bypass surgery.

Glenda and I, as well as my doctor, were very happy with the

results: I lost weight from about 270 to 210 pounds; my blood

sugar stabilized, and I could discontinue all diabetic medicines;

my sleep apnea abated and I no longer needed to sleep with a CPAP machine. There was only one occasional problem, and that was that sometimes at night I would have acid reflux, and a bit of food would come back up and then go back down through my trachea (often called windpipe) into my lungs. This aspiration could cause pneumonia severe enough to require antibiotics to conquer it. Before April of 2013 I experienced aspiration pneumonia a couple of times, and each time my doctor prescribed antibiotics to knock it out. Generally, however, I was able to avoid aspiration problems by having light dinners in the early evening, and making sure I didn't eat anything else later that night. But around the time of my birthday on April 7, 2013, I had enough acid reflux one evening to make me think I had possibly aspirated some food, so I saw my doctor, who prescribed ten days of the antibiotic Augmentin (amoxicillin) to ward off any possible pneumonia.

I took the Augmentin for eight days, then discontinued it because I didn't have any symptoms of pneumonia. I was troubled instead with what seemed a very mild case of diarrhea, for which I took the usual medicine, loperamide, the generic form of Imodium. At first the loperamide seemed effective, and I felt that I had things under good control and could continue with a plan I had to leave my home in Birmingham, Alabama and drive to visit friends in central Texas. I departed on April 18, a Thursday, little dreaming what lay in store for me. I arrived in Austin the next day, Friday, April 19, and began visiting several friends, making my Austin motel room my "headquarters." Over the next few days the mild diarrhea continued, however, and then began to worsen. I continued visiting friends, but had to go to the bathroom with increasing frequency. When traveling alone, I routinely call Glenda at least once each day, and by Wednesday, April 24 I told her when I called that I thought it wise to cut my visit a bit short and hit the road for home. I had visits planned with three different friends on the next day (the 25th), and said that I would keep those visits, then leave for home early on the morning of Friday, April 26 rather than Sunday, April 28 as originally planned. When I said I imagined I would have to make frequent bathroom stops on the drive home, and that I was a bit

worried that I might have "accidents" of diarrhea, Glenda
suggested that it might be a good idea to buy some adult diapers.
I found that idea rather embarrassing, but I also realized it was
sensible, so I bought some.

On Thursday, April 25, I drove from Austin down to New
Braunfels to see a longtime friend and classmate from high
school. We had lunch together, and I carefully ordered, not
wishing to dine on anything that I thought might exacerbate my
growing problem. Then I returned to Austin and visited a friend
from my graduate school days at the University of Texas-Austin.
By now I was not feeling very good. My friend asked if I wanted
to see her physician, but I declined. I told her I would go to my
motel, retire soon, and depart for home early the next morning.
When I got to my motel, I called and canceled a planned dinner
with another Austin friend. Then I took some more loperamide,
and went to bed. Though I had to visit the bathroom on several
occasions during the night, I managed to get some rest. Aware
that I could be getting dehydrated, I drank quite a bit of water.

Friday morning I arose around 4 a.m., went to the

bathroom, and then went to the front desk to check out and get my receipt. My legs felt heavy and I didn't feel as though I had very much strength. Nonetheless I loaded my small pickup truck and was about to leave when I realized that I hadn't put on a diaper. So I parked the truck and went back through the motel lobby to the motel's public men's room, concealing a diaper in a plastic grocery bag. After donning the diaper, I went back through the lobby to the truck and pulled out of the lot. I headed north on I-35 to Round Rock, where I turned east on US Highway 79. Birmingham lay about 780 miles distant. I filled my gas tank at one of the little towns along the highway, and kept driving eastward. I have driven all the way home on this route from Austin in one day before, but I decided that today I would just keep driving and see how I felt as I went along. I passed through several small towns I'd passed through many times before— Taylor, Rockdale, Hearne, Buffalo, Palestine, Jacksonville, Henderson, and several others, leaving US 79 in Henderson to take Texas highway 43 to Marshall, where I got on I-20, eastbound. In retrospect, I am sure I had no business driving as I did, feeling as I did, but I truly did not realize just how sick I was getting, and the homing instinct is strong.

After I entered Louisiana and passed through Shreveport, I stopped at an Interstate rest stop around 12:30 in the afternoon. I called Glenda and told her where I was. I said I didn't feel so hot and didn't have an appetite, so I was going to take a nap. I told her I would travel on after the nap, stopping at a motel overnight, then coming on home the next day. I added that I would call her again when I stopped for the night. I couldn't know it at the time, but that would be the last call I made to Glenda that day. After the call, I slouched in the driver's seat, closed my eyes, and dozed. I don't know how long I slept, but I was awakened by a gentle knocking on my windshield. A man was checking to see if I was all right. I shot him a smile and a thumb's up, and he returned my smile and waved as he headed toward his car. I stretched, went in to the rest stop bathroom, and then resumed my eastward travel on I-20—Minden, Arcadia, Grambling, Ruston, and as I approached Monroe, I was unaware of what time it was. Perhaps it was 4 p.m., perhaps 5, but I remember thinking that Monroe was well over half of the way home, and that I could use some more rest. After passing through most of Monroe, I pulled off the Interstate and checked in at a motel. I wasn't hungry and had no plan to eat; by now I had decided that anything I ate or drank would just go right through me, anyway.

My memories of my night in the motel room are few but vivid. I recall finding my room and going inside, putting my overnight duffle and shaving bags on the bed, and sitting down on a small couch to watch television. I don't remember what I was watching. I do remember that the diarrhea started again, and this time I was completely powerless to stop it. It was relentless. My stool was leaking onto the couch, but I was unable to get up when I realized what was happening. Later—and I have no idea how much later it was—I managed to get up off the couch and go into the bathroom, noticing that I had stool in and on my jeans, my socks, my sneakers. I was not thinking coherently at all. I remember getting into the bathtub with the vague idea of cleaning myself up, but I still wore my jeans, socks, and sneakers. I slipped around in the tub and had trouble getting up. I don't know how I got out of the tub, but still later, I found myself on the motel room floor in front of the television, too weak to get up. Yet even later, I was conscious that it was morning. (This was Saturday, April 27.) I somehow found my cell phone and called Glenda, who was greatly relieved to hear from me—she had been trying to reach me since about 4 o'clock the previous afternoon, when she thought she'd check on me and see where I was. In my condition I had completely forgotten I had told her I'd call her when I stopped for the night. I was still very weak and not thinking very straight.

"Where are you?" she asked.

"I don't know," I replied. "Wait a minute and I'll check and let you know," I said, and then, much to her consternation (I later learned), I hung up. I don't know how long it took me to find the plastic card that was also my room key and which bore the name and phone number of my motel. Once I located it, I called Glenda back and gave her the name of my motel and my room number.

"You're in trouble," she said, and I was in no condition to

disagree. She said she was going to call the front desk, explain the situation, and have them call an ambulance. Not long after I hung up, I heard a knock. I managed to get to the door and open it before falling on the floor yet again. Two or three EMTs entered. One said, "What's wrong?"

"I have diarrhea," I replied.

Exaggerating a sniff, he said "I can tell *that*," but I was too sick to feel insulted or even embarrassed. I felt relief for the help I was beginning to get because clearly nothing I had tried in the last 24 or so hours had availed. The EMT crew then loaded me into the ambulance and took me to Monroe's St. Francis Medical Center. I was conscious during the transit, and directed an EMT man to my wallet, where I always carry an emergency information card which gives my name, whom to contact, and a list of all my medications and dosages, including not only prescription medicines but also over-the-counter medicines.

GLENDA:

Looking in the rear view mirror that time affords, I can see that our nightmare adventure began innocuously enough. It crept up on our blind side, did its damage, and left us with some lessons for the future, as well as an overwhelming sense of gratitude to all those who helped us. As he notes above, Ralph had been susceptible to aspiration pneumonia for several years. When he aspirated a bit of food sometime during the second week of April, he experienced a bit of fever, and, because he had a trip scheduled for the next week, decided to see his doctor. He didn't want a case of pneumonia in the first place, and he also didn't want to cancel his long-planned trip to Austin. In response to his complaint, our internist prescribed an antibiotic that Ralph took for several days until he began to experience slight diarrhea, at which point he decided after 8 days, rather than the 10 prescribed, to discontinue the medicine because he was experiencing no signs of pneumonia. When he left for Austin, he felt pretty good.

Ralph has always loved the open road, and, once or twice a year has traveled by himself to visit friends in various parts of the United States. He is a good driver, and I've welcomed his traveling alone as a prime time for my daughter, Betsy, to visit from Orlando to do mother-daughter things with me here in Birmingham. I had invited her for this occasion. She and I were shopping at one of our area malls when, on Wednesday, April 26, at 12:38 p.m. (a precise time that will always live in my memory bank) my antiquated, flip-top cell phone rang. I knew that Ralph was on his way home; he had been in touch once or twice a day while he was away, but this time he called to say he was feeling "punk," and would probably stop somewhere along the way and resume his trip home tomorrow. I said, "I love you," and "keep me posted." I told Betsy about the phone call, and we resumed our shopping. I was a little worried because of the continual—but apparently controllable—diarrhea that he had experienced during the trip.

The phone call and his description of "feeling punk" prompted increasing concern, especially when, after a couple of hours, I began trying to reach him by cell phone to assure myself that all was okay. No answer. I called again and again and again.

No answer. After leaving the mall, Betsy and I dropped by a neighborhood restaurant for a bite of supper, and returned home for the evening. I tried Ralph's number dozens of times. Still no answer. Betsy and I began checking the weather report for areas along I-20, Ralph's route home, and learned that heavy rain was expected. Betsy tried to reassure me that Ralph had probably checked into a room for the night; he might, she said, have left his cell phone in the truck, and, because of the wet weather and his crummy condition, had not returned to the truck to collect it. That assuaged my feelings a bit but not enough to prevent my trying to reach him throughout the evening. My worry grew. I longed for a "smart" phone so that he—and his phone—could easily be located. Later in the evening, when I called AT&T to ask what could be done to locate his cell phone, technicians informed me that, because the phone was in his name, I must have his permission to tamper with the account in any way. I clearly couldn't make that happen, so I circumvented the difficulty in a follow-up phone call by giving the technician Ralph's social security number. She then instructed me in downloading a program that could help. Unfortunately, and for reasons I don't understand, I could not complete the download until about 3 a.m. the next day.

After a night of fitful sleep, awaking often to check my computer for the cell-phone-location download, I woke up around 3 a.m. to discover that Ralph's cell phone had been tracked to Monroe, Louisiana near the Pecan Land Mall. Foolishly, but hopefully, I tried his number several more times. No luck. I called the Monroe Police Department to ask them to drive around motel parking lots in the area to see if they could locate his white Tacoma truck. No help there. Ralph was not yet "missing" by police definition. Finally, around 7 a.m. or so, I called Ralph's eldest son, John, who lives in Knoxville, Tennessee, to tell him that his dad was missing and that the police were unable or unwilling to help. While the two of us discussed a plan whereby we could call all motels in the area, my land line beeped. It was Ralph calling me!

I immediately asked Ralph, "Where are you?" When he told me he didn't know, I knew something was badly amiss. He said he would find out, but, much to my dismay, he hung up the phone. I don't recall whether I successfully reached him on a return call, or whether he called me back. Nonetheless, when we reconnected, he was able to tell me he was at the Comfort Suites in Monroe, Louisiana, and he gave me the motel's phone number. I immediately called the front desk and told the receptionist that my husband was in a room there, was "in trouble," and needed an ambulance. She told me in a return phone call that the ambulance was taking him to St. Francis Memorial Hospital.

After updating John, who was preparing to alert his brothers (Walker and Collin), Betsy and I made some hasty decisions. We would drive in my car to Monroe (thank God she was here in Birmingham with me), and once we arrived there she would do a quick turnaround to drive Ralph's truck back to Birmingham. Doing so would give her transportation back to Birmingham (where she would return Ralph's truck to our garage and be able to catch her flight to Orlando the next day) and, at the same time, allow me to have just one vehicle in Louisiana.

I threw enough clothes for a couple of days into a bag,

grabbed my I-pad and cell phone, spotted our neighbor, Bill Odom, near his driveway and hastily asked him to look after things, then Betsy and I headed west. I drove about as fast as I thought the law and safety would allow. Betsy kept offering to drive, but I felt I had to be actively doing something to get us there. I have little memory of what Betsy and I talked about other than trying to make the best decision about whether to go first to the hospital or to Comfort Suites. Because the 355 mile drive from our home to Monroe is about 5½ hours, we reasoned that it would be best to go first to the motel so that Betsy could hop in the pickup for her return trip to Birmingham. I was afraid that a trip to the hospital could result in a long delay for Betsy.

As we drove west along I-20, I had Betsy calling information for important phone numbers. First among them was information on how to reach the Emergency Room of St. Francis Memorial Hospital. She called the number and handed me the phone. After I explained who and where I was, the operator connected me with the nurse who was assisting Ralph. The nurse very patiently explained that he was taking care of "a very sick man." I asked him to tell Ralph that I was on my way, and gave him my cell number. Some minutes later, my cell phone rang. It was an emergency-room doctor from St. Francis who explained that this was "scary stuff," if, indeed, Ralph's tests proved what he strongly suspected: *Clostridium difficile*.

The car and my thoughts were racing. I knew that the doctor was warning me that this was serious business; I had heard about super-bugs but actually knew very little about them, especially this one. Despite the doctor's tone and my subsequent sense of worry that the worst could happen, I also entertained thoughts that Ralph would be in the hospital just a few days, and then released to travel back to Birmingham. Betsy was a real moral support, putting the best face on things, and encouraging me to be positive. She used my iPad to find directions to Comfort Suites, and we went directly there once we were in Monroe. We pulled into the parking lot, and I spotted Ralph's truck and remarked to Betsy, "He's really sick; look how crookedly he parked." She already knew that Ralph is a stickler for parking "between the lines," and his truck was definitely over the lines.

We entered the motel building and checked with the receptionist, who took us to what had been Ralph's room. The minute we opened the door we realized this was no ordinary diarrhea; the stench was horrid, enough so that we immediately recognized it as septic. We found Ralph's keys, and I walked Betsy to the truck, hugged her, and sent her on her way back to Birmingham. She still had the 5 ½ hour return trip ahead of her. Not until she left did I realize I had assigned her to a vehicle that was likely germ-infested. I learned later, with relief, that she, too, had considered the germs and wisely decided to drink only a milkshake to avoid handling food that she would be putting in her mouth.

20 Days in Monroe

RALPH:

When you're riding in the back of an ambulance with an EMT monitoring your blood pressure (mine was very low), your heart rate (ditto), and other vital signs, you don't notice anything about the neighborhoods through which you're passing. Everything seems surreal; you're conscious that you're the patient headed toward the hospital, but it's hard to wrap your head around the fact that it's *you* on the gurney, *you* whose vital signs are being monitored, *you* who is obviously the one in trouble. We arrived at the hospital's emergency entrance, and I was transferred inside. I don't know how much time passed before I found myself in the hospital's Critical Care Unit (CCU), but I do remember a very good nurse who was in authority. I had a nasty scrape high on my forehead, probably caused when I fell and my head hit the tightly-woven carpet in the motel room. I had a similar scrape on my right shoulder. I also had a wide assortment of bruises—something I often had, especially on my hands and arms—thanks to taking doctor-advised frequent low doses of aspirin. Of paramount importance, however, was that I had been having an almost constant flow of diarrhea, and my legs and mid-section were grotesquely swollen, what the nurse in charge called "severe edema."

I began to feel embarrassed because no matter how I tried to hold the diarrhea, I was utterly unsuccessful. Doctors seemed to swarm around me as I was hooked up to an intravenous (IV) device supplying fluids and medicines to me. I recall speaking with one of the doctors, who, I later learned, was the one who had called Glenda while she was on her way to Monroe. He had a very pleasant manner and asked me what I did for a living. I said I was a retired English professor. He asked who my favorite poet is, and I told him there are many I like, but one of my favorites is William Wordsworth, some of whose lines have "echoed" in my mind for many years. Thereafter, whenever I saw him, he called me "Professor." Among other doctors were a nephrologist, present because my kidneys had more or less stopped functioning; and a gastroenterologist, doubtless there because of the persistent diarrhea. Yet another doctor was present. I know each doctor spoke with me, but I don't recall specifics of what they said. Not long after they left, the nurse in charge came back.

What the nurse in charge had was some sort of waste management device designed to carry off my stool through a tube to a plastic bag and thus save nurses and their aides the task of repeatedly changing my diapers. The device had to be inserted in my rectum, and the nurse successfully installed it after some difficulty with me, for the process was painful. "I know this hurts," she explained, "but it will make things better." The presence of the device meant I could not lie directly on my back, but rather I had to lie tilted toward one side or the other, so that the tube carrying away my frequent wastes would not be crimped or clogged. Because I was perpetually weak, uncomfortable, and unable to shift myself in the bed, I often pushed the call button and asked to be turned from lying on one side to lying on the other. A word of fact here, not necessarily a word of complaint: If you're in a hospital bed and need attention, pushing the call button is not necessarily going to get you quick relief. After you

push the button, a voice will respond: "How may I help you?"
You then say what you want, a message that draws such
responses as "I'll tell your nurse," "I'll send someone," or words
to that effect—but then you may lie there for quite a long time
until someone actually comes. The delay, of course, can be for
several perfectly good reasons; you're not, after all, the only
patient being cared for. But I wouldn't be truthful if I said that I
got satisfactory responses in all instances of my pushing the call
button in all three of my hospitalizations resulting from my C.
diff infections. I will say that during my hospitalization in
Monroe responses to my calls were generally satisfactory—for
which I am grateful. (It strikes me as somewhat strangely
reflective of hospital hierarchy to note that when referring to
nurses, we generally use their first names, but when referring to
doctors, we generally refer to their last names, preceded, of
course, by "Dr." I regret that I can't remember the last names of
most of my nurses.)

As I lay in my bed someone—perhaps one of the nurses—
told me that a doctor had spoken on the phone with Glenda, who

was on her way to Monroe. I later found out that Glenda's

daughter, Betsy McClain, who was visiting from Florida, was

coming with her. I don't know how long it took Glenda and Betsy

to get to Monroe; all I remember is that I was glad Glenda was

coming, even though it seemed more or less to prove to me that I

really was seriously ill. I dozed fitfully between watching

television shows. Re-runs of "The Golden Girls" and

"Gunsmoke" seemed to run together when they had nothing in

common. The terrorist bombing of the Boston Marathon

dominated the news. Years and years ago, when I was a

freshman in college, a man named Newton Minow famously

described television as a "vast wasteland." He wasn't wrong then,

and his words still seem to me to ring with considerable truth.

Aside from the news, there wasn't much on TV that I found

interesting, and there is no drag-by time like hospital drag-by

time. And because I was virtually an invalid, I could barely

move. Ironically, powerlessness is a powerful feeling.

GLENDA:

Once the motel receptionist gave me directions to the hospital, and I had secured my own room for the night, I left to find Ralph. I found him, as directed, in the Critical Care Unit of the hospital, and, with his flushed cheeks, he looked deceptively healthy. I had not yet noticed his enormously swollen abdomen and legs. The various tubes and monitors, however, were enough to tell me that this was serious business, reinforcing what his nurses and doctors attending him were reporting. Over the next several days, I was to learn a lot about C. diff.

One of my first lessons in the disease came from our internist. On Monday, following Ralph's admission to the hospital in Monroe on Saturday, I called her office and reported to her receptionist what had happened to Ralph. That evening, around 9 p.m., shortly after I had settled into my room for the evening, I received a call from our internist, expressing concern for what had happened. Her compassion was heart warming, and her overview of the disease helped me realize what we were in for. I listened carefully to what the various doctors at St. Francis told me, but, as many patients and their family members can attest, listening when in stress leaves one with more questions than answers. And so I used my time—those long hours in the Critical Care Unit waiting room—to learn as much as I could about C. diff and the pseudo membranous colitis and rhabdomyolysis besetting him. (Rhabdomyolysis is a disintegration of muscle, associated with excretion of myoglobin in the urine, frequently seen with severe diarrhea)

My iPad proved invaluable as I searched the Internet, what *Good Housekeeping* has called the "doctor of the desperate." (November 2013, p. 103.) I googled the Mayo Clinic website and learned that C. diff is, among medical professionals, more accurately known as *Clostridium difficile*, a devastating bacterium that has in recent years become more prevalent, causing severe and watery diarrhea and/or colon inflammation. Severe cases require hospitalization because patients become dehydrated, can experience kidney failure, weight loss, increased white blood cell count, and blood poisoning. I learned there and elsewhere that the use of antibiotics often precedes the development of C. diff. Antibiotics can destroy good bacteria in the gut and allow the toxic bacteria to flourish. Indeed, according to the Mayo Clinic website, "even mild to moderate *C. difficile* infections can quickly progress to a fatal disease if not treated promptly." (www.mayoclinic.org/diseases-conditions/c-difficile/basics/definition/con-20029664.)

Ralph had most of the characteristic symptoms, and he had, of course, been on antibiotics. It became clear, in fact, that his dehydration and septic condition had prompted a dramatic and dangerous drop in blood pressure, explaining why he had spent much of the previous night on the floor where he had fallen, indifferent to the sound of his ringing phone, and unable to seek the help he needed. On my initial visit the day of my arrival to the hospital, I did not yet understand how he had gotten those wounds on his head and arm, carpet abrasions from his motel room that were, at the moment, the least of our concerns, but that have left minor scars telling their own story of a night of horror.

Ralph was scheduled to appear on the program of the

32nd annual William Inge Theatre Festival, an event he had attended for most of its 32 year history. May 1-4, 2013 were particularly important dates, representing as they did the 100th anniversary of the playwright Inge's birth in Independence, Kansas. A native Kansan, Ralph has through much of his educational experience been interested in Inge, a fellow Kansan, and eventually in 1989 published a biography on him. Thus, he has always been on the program during the Festival week. While sitting in the waiting room, I read an email from Peter Ellenstein, the Festival Director, with a reminder about the upcoming program. I responded to Peter, telling him of Ralph's hospitalization and the need for us to cancel our trip to Independence. Thus began a series of emails not only to Peter and other Inge acquaintances, but also to family and friends.

The list of recipients grew as very kind and solicitous people began to inquire about Ralph, offering all kinds of help—hugs and prayers, thoughts and notes. I unabashedly encouraged folks to send cards, and they came pouring in. I cannot overestimate the role all those gestures played in the healing process. While flowers are welcome, too many of them can crowd a room, but kind thoughts of relatives and friends can fill the mind with many reasons for getting well. Visitors, too, brought comfort. Most important among them were Ralph's three sons. John came from Knoxville; Walker came from Hays, Kansas; and Collin came from Tuscaloosa. Because Collin has a night job, his mom, Karen, took a day from work on April 30 to drive Collin to Monroe to see his dad. Collin could get his sleep while his mom drove, and, therefore, be rested enough to return to work for his night shift. Ralph and Karen raised three very fine sons, and I cannot say enough about how much their visits meant to their dad.

My husband is not known for patience, but I was touched by how hour after hour he lay on his back—or on whatever part of his back could endure the discomfort—and patiently did his part toward trying not only to survive, but, eventually, to get well enough to go home. His was a grit that on any other occasion I might call "intestinal fortitude," but here that description seems too clever by far. To help pass the day-upon-day of waiting for healing, and to lift his spirits, I would read him the notes friends had sent, and show him the pictures young nieces and nephews had drawn for him.

RALPH:

As far as I knew, I didn't have a diagnosis yet as I lay fitfully in my Critical Care Unit bed at St. Francis Medical Center in Monroe. I underwent a multitude of tests, scans, blood samplings, you-name-it. I later learned that the doctors suspected a "super-bug," probably C. diff, but I don't remember anyone telling me that at first. I was so glad to see Glenda come walking into the room that I temporarily ignored my discomfort. By this time I knew I was really sick and therefore in the right place, but I still didn't know just *how* sick. Glenda did not betray the worry I know she was feeling; she tried to be upbeat as she told me that she and Betsy had arrived at the motel where I had stayed. She kidded me about how poorly I had parked my truck at the motel, and said that she had checked in to that motel and would continue to stay there while I was hospitalized. Betsy, who had a plane to catch from Birmingham to her home in Orlando the next day, had left, driving my pickup home. Glenda had let my three sons and my six sisters know what had happened and where I was. I don't remember how long it was before all three of my sons and their mother, and three of my sisters and a brother-in-law, all came to see me at the hospital in Monroe.

Not long after my hospitalization in Monroe, Glenda combed our computer's e-mail address book and began informing relatives and friends far and wide about my situation; as a result I began receiving countless messages expressing get-well wishes and prayers from so many people to whom I am deeply grateful. Hospital employees said they'd never seen so many cards come for a patient; Glenda daily brought get-well cards to me, and also read to me the many get-well e-mails she had received.

The nephrologist told me that though I needed dialysis, he thought there was a good chance that my kidney function would return. The idea of dialysis sobered me significantly; I had friends who were getting dialysis three or four times each week, and I knew it was a very serious matter. Moreover, one of the other doctors told me that I might need surgery to remove my colon, meaning I would have a colectomy and thus spend the rest of my days disposing of my waste in a throw-away bag. I seized on the nephrologist's optimism about my kidney function returning and the other doctor's use of the word *might* when he mentioned a colectomy. One of the CCU nurses put it most succinctly when she told me she didn't think I realized how sick I was. What the doctors had said pressed that point home. I am not a demonstratively religious person, but I remember taking Glenda's hand and saying to her, "Pray for me."

GLENDA:

I developed a routine toward making the Comfort Suites my temporary home. It was several days, however, before I asked the staff what they planned to do with the room Ralph had occupied. "No way," I said, "can you rent out that room." I knew that the septic smell would be next to impossible to clear away, and by now I also knew enough to worry about the C. diff spores that were no doubt thriving in that space. I was greatly relieved to learn that the room had been isolated and that the extensive remodeling project going on in the motel had not yet reached that section of the hallway. Carpets, draperies, and furnishings were all scheduled to be replaced anyway—a lucky coincidence. On my second day in Monroe, I had removed Ralph's belongings from his room, had thrown away shoes, jeans, and other clothing that were infected beyond redemption. I had bought a bottle of chlorine bleach that I kept in my room, and had scrubbed his wallet, watch, and other items that aren't normally subjected to such harsh abrasion.

The staff at Comfort Suites were especially kind, inquiring each day how Ralph was. Each morning I ate breakfast there, and at night I could do my laundry in the bathroom sink, making do with the few clothes I had brought. Not until the second week did I decide I needed at least one more change of clothing and a second pair of pajamas. The mall was not far away, but I made a hurried trip there because I felt pressed for time, grabbing what I could readily find that would meet my needs. I ate lunch each day in the hospital cafeteria, except for those welcome occasions when Ralph had family visitors who would join me for lunch away from the hospital. I returned to my room late each day, where I would set up a food tray and eat whatever fast food I had picked up. I usually closed out each day by sending emails to friends, or talking on the phone with them.

RALPH:

It's hard to express the gratitude I felt when other family came to see me and offer their love and support for Glenda and me. John, my oldest son, who lives in Knoxville with my daughter-in-law Jennifer and their two children Alexandra and Zachary, had arrived not long after Glenda. He said he thought "the Man upstairs" had been looking out for me, and given my gradual realization that I could well have perished in that motel room, I believed he was right. Walker, my middle son, who has a nursing degree and lives in Hays, Kansas, arrived soon after, telling me that his GPS had given him a route that took him through countless small north-Texas towns with one or two stoplights. I couldn't explain his GPS to him, but I appreciated his immediate take-care-of-medical-business approach. He asked doctors knowledgeable questions about my white-cell counts (as high as 43,000 at one point, according to one of the mass email "bulletins" that Glenda sent out and that I examined later), heart rate and other vital matters that were being monitored daily, and reassured me that I was in good hands.

On Tuesday, April 30, Walker wrote to his friends in the medical community in Hays, Kansas:

Just spoke with the CCU doc. Dad remains in critical condition. However, the doc is pleased with his small steps forward. The good news is his white blood cell count is down to 28,000. Yesterday the doc said he would be elated if it were down to 35,000 today, given the overwhelming infection and the level of shock he sustained. That was certainly welcome news. He is on a BiPap (respiratory support) full time but hasn't required a ventilator. That is encouraging because the doc believed that Dad was very close to needing that on Sunday. However, as Dad took a step forward on one front, he took one back from a lung aspect. He has accumulated some fluid in the lungs. They will attempt to remove the fluid with the dialysis currently in process. He may still require mechanical ventilation. Acute Respiratory Distress is the concern but so far been avoided. All of his organs took a tremendous blow from the septic shock he experienced. There are too many potential concerns to list but Dad remains awake and responsive. He's tired but fighting, and the fact he's still here is a testament to his strength and the care and love he is getting.

It is probably a good thing that at the time I didn't realize just how bad my medical situation was.

Also on April 30, Collin, my youngest son, arrived with Karen, my ex-wife (also a nurse), both of whom live in Tuscaloosa. Collin works nights, and Karen had graciously taken the day off and driven him over during the morning while he slept, then drove him back to Tuscaloosa so that he could work that night. Collin's message was firm: Do what the doctors tell you to do, stay strong, and fight this thing; believe you're going to get better. He earnestly repeated a line from the poet Dylan Thomas to me: "Do not go gentle into that good night." I just about lost it then, for quoting poetry is not something I expected from Collin. The intensity of his feeling touched me somewhere very deep inside.

The diagnosis of C. diff came fairly soon after I was hospitalized in Monroe when the gastroenterologist performed a sigmoidoscopy, an examination of my colon. The doctors ordered treatments that included oral doses of Vancomycin, Flagyl, and other medicines, and periodic dialysis. However, the diarrhea remained persistent during this treatment, though one bright spot was that the nephrologist repeatedly told me he thought my kidneys had a very good chance to recover. After a few more days of treatment, the persistence of the diarrhea caused the gastroenterologist to order another examination of my colon. By this time my sisters Betty, Alice, and Marilyn were in Monroe, along with Earl, Alice's husband, who drove them down from their homes in Kansas. After the gastroenterologist's inspection, he told Glenda I had "a raging case of C. diff." The doctors decided to try treating the C. diff with Vancomycin enemas every six hours. After that, I had many enemas of that medicine, and I seem to recall also taking oral doses. Neither treatment was particularly effective; the collection bag of the waste-disposal device in my fanny continued to get filled from diarrhea.

Still, there were encouraging things: At the nurses' and physical therapists' urging, I was able to get out of bed (with their assistance) and sit in a chair for awhile, despite my fanny being so sore from the waste elimination device. I also no longer needed intravenous nutrition; everything I ate was by mouth. I favored orange sherbet; however, I deplored the protein shakes the nurses constantly encouraged me to down. I thought they tasted just awful. They accumulated on my bedside tray because they were left in hopes I'd eventually down them. I tried a few times, because I knew I needed protein, but for the most part I couldn't stand their taste.

Meanwhile, my kidneys were still too sluggish to do their job, so I continued to have periodic dialysis, which at first took place right in my CCU room, administered by a young woman who spoke little. It was a lengthy process during which I tried to find something interesting on television—a largely fruitless task. I do remember the last dialysis I had in my CCU room. It was administered by an older man who was about to go out of town for a couple of weeks. As I understood him, he was a traveling dialysis technician, and it was time for him to hit the road to another hospital. Before he left, though, he said he knew that the nephrologist was optimistic that my kidney function would return. "I think you're going to be okay," he told me; "I'm going to remember you and pray for you." Here was a stranger who wasn't witnessing to me or sermonizing in any way; he was just simply saying he cared and that he would pray. It is an example, to borrow a famous line from Tennessee Williams, of "the kindness of strangers," a kindness that recurred many times during my struggle.

I mentioned earlier that I am not a particularly religious man in the sense that I am a regular churchgoer who subscribes to a particular organized church denomination's stated beliefs. I am, however, a man of feeling, one who sees and appreciates all of creation with a sense of wonder and respect. My upbringing included Sunday-school teachings in the Nazarene and Methodist denominations, and my literary training included a wide range of writings that express human spirituality in a variety of ways. Lying in my CCU bed, I could look out a window to my right and see the green, waxy leaves of a magnolia tree through the opened blinds. A bit farther on, past the magnolia leaves, I could see a small stone cross atop a building. I would occasionally focus on that cross, and came to see it as a kind of talisman, symbolic that somehow, some way, I was going to get better. The thing to do was abide, follow the doctors' orders, hope, and cling to my sense that I would pull through.

On Thursday, May 9—eleven days after my initial hospitalization in Monroe--I was moved from the CCU to what the hospital employees called a "step-down" room. I no longer needed the kind of crisis-level care that the CCU was for, though of course I was still very ill and was still stuck in my bed. I welcomed the change of rooms, and I could now see that the magnolia tree I referred to earlier was in a courtyard, and Glenda told me that there were also flowers in the courtyard below. I couldn't see the small stone cross anymore, but I knew it was still there, and I took some comfort in that knowledge. By now I was continuing to receive enemas of Vancomycin, but all my symptoms, including the diarrhea and swelling of my legs and abdomen, persisted. I was now being taken for dialysis to a room where several other patients were on dialysis.

GLENDA:

The email responses from friends, as well as their phone calls, gave me gossipy tidbits to share with Ralph each morning. Our main conversation, however, was focused on going home from the hospital. It was a driving force for both Ralph and me, but if we wanted to go home, Ralph had to be well enough to be dismissed from the hospital. That wasn't happening, although he had improved enough by May 9 to leave the Critical Care Unit and go to what hospital personnel called the "step-down" unit. Meantime, three of Ralph's sisters and a brother-in-law had come from Kansas for a visit. They were as interested as I in knowing his white blood cell count (WBC), a question I posed first thing each morning when I arrived at the hospital. That blood count was like unreliable spring weather: fickle. I never knew whether the news would be encouraging or discouraging, but that daily report was a barometer for telling a layperson like me what was happening regarding Ralph's C. diff infection, and how long before we could depart for home. In fact, his WBC was sometimes as high as 43,000; other days, we were encouraged by a lower number, only to be disappointed the very next day when it would have spiked again. (A normal WBC range is between 4,500 and 10,000 cells per cubic millimeter). The day following Ralph's move to the step down unit (May 10), Ralph's gastroenterologist ordered another sigmoidoscopy to check for the persistence of the C. diff. For this procedure, the surgeon inserted a flexible tube, connected to a fiber optic camera, into the rectum and sigmoid colon looking for traces of the disease. The report came back: He still had a raging case of C. diff. Ralph's visiting family members—Betty, Alice, Marilyn, and Earl—were sitting beside me when the doctor broke the news. I burst into tears, but felt especially glad that they were there. I would have felt so alone otherwise.

Meantime, Ralph and I behaved much like E.T. from the Spielberg movie of 1982 in our longing to go home. St Francis had been wonderful, but being 355 miles away from home when life is hanging in the balance is not where you want to be. True, I was embraced by others in the CCU waiting room, other people like me who had family members who might not make it. While there, I rediscovered how important the kindness of strangers can be. The waiting room was the great leveler; beneath the friendly chatter we were all caring for each other as members of a human race that had forgotten divisions of black and white, the well-heeled and the poorly shod. But these persons, despite their own concerns for loved ones, asked each day how my husband was faring and communicated their understanding of our need to get home. I will never forget how I felt embraced by these strangers' concerns, and the sense of community and caring established in that CCU waiting room.

RALPH:

I don't remember whether it was during my first or my second dialysis after my move to the step-down room that a doctor I didn't recognize spoke to me and said he thought that a fecal transplant could work to restore my health. "But they don't do fecal transplants here," he said, citing a policy decision made by the hospital's administration. He must also have mentioned fecal transplants to Glenda, or perhaps some other doctors did, for it wasn't long after that when she began to study fecal transplants on the internet and to make other inquiries. Her first mention of it in one of her daily "health bulletin" emails sent out to friends came on May 11, after the doctor had made his morning visit. Glenda wrote that the doctor had "expressed some willingness to try a fecal implant if that seems a suitable plan of action." The next day she wrote in her daily "bulletin" email, "Alabama friends: do you know of a hospital in Birmingham that does fecal transplants? They don't do them here, I was told this morning." Fecal transplants were more or less considered experimental by the Federal Food and Drug Administration (FDA), and perhaps it was partly for that reason that they were not performed at Monroe's St. Francis Medical Center; I don't know. I didn't give it a lot of thought at first, but I didn't know at the time how much Glenda was making a point of finding out more.

GLENDA:

Regulations became a barrier to going home. We learned that changing hospitals was not an easy option. Insurance regulations stipulate that to move between hospitals requires that the receiving hospital provide a service that the dismissing hospital is unable to provide. Ralph's medical team included a gastroenterologist, a nephrologist, a surgeon, a cardiologist. What additional services could we possibly want?

What we wanted was a fecal transplant, a procedure I had been researching because of a suggestion by a nephrology assistant who thought Ralph might be a candidate. At about the same time, Sandra, one of my two sisters, told me about a friend of hers, whom I scarcely knew. This friend, she said, had taken an unusual interest in Ralph's case. Indeed, the friend's story provided a poignant backdrop for our understanding her stake in what was happening to Ralph. Several years ago, this friend's husband had suffered from a serious C. diff infection. Their daughter had at that time researched fecal transplants and had asked her dad's doctors about performing one, but they said it was not available. The husband subsequently died from C. diff complications. But Sandra's friend felt that she had valuable information that could help Ralph, and, this time, intervening on our behalf, pointed us in a direction that she thought might save my husband. Because she let us know about the potential of fecal transplants for saving lives, we owe her much credit for what was to follow.

RALPH:

Meanwhile, as Glenda did her iPad research, my drag-by hospital time continued. I lay tilted to first one side, then the other, alternately watched television and dozed, and was frequently awakened for routine matters like giving me medicine, drawing blood, checking my vital signs, or bringing me food. Rest seemed to have little to do with my lying there in that hospital bed. Television continued to be mostly poor entertainment; I paid fitful attention to old episodes of "The Golden Girls," "Seinfeld," and current shows like "The Voice" and "Survivor," but took no serious interest. One Sunday night I watched what was, I gathered, a two-hour "season finale" of "Survivor." Supposedly a "reality show," "Survivor" involved a group of people going through various sorts of programmed duress on a tropical island. These people were contestants, and only one of them would eventually prevail (though the losers didn't die, so the title of the show is clearly hype). I watched it fully aware that I certainly didn't have to, but there was something about the irony of the situation that preoccupied me: The people on the so-called "reality show" were battling to win a contest with a phony survival theme, while I was lying sick in the hospital, and I was the one who was trying *really* to survive. Emotions can run high, unpredictable, and contradictory when you're lying gravely ill for hours in a hospital bed; I couldn't pay serious attention to the "Survivor" television episode, but on another night, however, the Turner Classic Movie channel featured an old black and white Jean Renoir film, *The Southerner*, a tale of a poor family's persistence in struggling to survive. The portrayal of their stubborn refusal to give up their struggle touched me. It was kind of over-the-top, but I took some heart from watching it, even though it, too, being a movie, could hardly be taken very seriously.

I don't remember when John and Walker went home, as did my sisters and brother-in-law. Collin, now with time off from his job, returned and took up residence with Achilles, his dog, in a motel near the motel where Glenda was staying. He is uncomfortable, as many people are, in hospitals; he didn't like waiting for the limited visiting times, and he always stood, rather than sitting, when he was in my room. His message remained constant: stay strong, believe, obey the doctors. Glenda kept me posted with the cards and other get-well messages sent by relatives and friends. The show of concern from others was deeply gratifying and very remarkable: one day, May 10, I received no less than 24 cards.

Lying with a sore fanny in a hospital bed can be frustrating because the discomfort tempts you to press the call button in a constant quest for relief that is just as constantly elusive. I tried not to be a pest, but there was no way I could lie that wouldn't begin to hurt after a short while. I was given pain pills, usually Lortab, which eased the pain somewhat, but those had to be spaced to respect their potency. Pills to help me sleep during the long nights were mostly ineffective. For one thing, as I mentioned earlier, if I happened to be asleep, I would often be awakened for a check of my vital signs. For another, blood had to be drawn frequently for testing; doctors were closely monitoring my blood's white and red cell counts. I've never been blasé about being "stuck" for a blood test; my veins are not obvious to all nurses, and let's face it: some nurses are better than others at finding a good vein to stick. I can't watch the puncturing, and I hate it—both for me and the nurse—when multiple sticks are needed to get the required amount of blood for testing. I had been catheterized, but I don't remember exactly when. Other matters of daily hygiene concerned me. I have a beard that I had previously kept neatly trimmed; normal care of my beard meant that I frequently had to shave and trim it to keep it shaped properly, but while hospitalized I could neither trim it nor shave without help, and although Collin did give me a shave at one point, I later learned that I shouldn't be shaved because a nick could cause bleeding and/or infection. I usually brush my teeth two or three times daily, and floss at least once a day, but all I was afforded while hospitalized was a small brush and a small tube of paste that at least allowed me to brush sporadically after a nurse or aide brought me some water and a "spit cup." I'm sure if I had insisted I could have brushed, even flossed, more often, but I didn't.

I was on a mostly-liquid diet—broth, jello, and those aforementioned chocolate-flavored protein drinks that I usually gagged on. My muscles were continuing to atrophy from lack of use, and though I knew I really needed protein, I just couldn't get those shakes down. Thank goodness for my orange sherbet and popsicles. And, of course, everything I ate still seemed to go right through me. I had no real appetite, and I lost weight rapidly. One day seemed to run into the next for me as I lay in the Monroe hospital. But Glenda was busily checking into fecal transplants and how I might be brought back home to Birmingham.

GLENDA:

Ralph and I now knew which treatment we wanted and began asking questions about getting the fecal transplant procedure done. At first, we thought that St. Francis could perform the transplant, but we learned that hospital protocol would not allow it. To my email friends, I sent out an "all points bulletin," asking where in Birmingham such a thing might be done. Most leads proved dead ends, complicated also by several factors, one because of the yuck factor; another because it is not a money-making procedure for hospitals or for drug companies either, explaining in part why it is rarely performed. I was warned about yet another obstacle by my son Johnny, with whom I spoke on the phone almost daily, and who works in one of our Birmingham area hospitals. On Monday, May 20th, he called and told me about the conversation he had just had with a gastroenterologist at his workplace. "Mom," he said, "don't expect to bring Ralph to Birmingham for a fecal transplant. Just this week, the FDA has ruled that they can no longer be done." Indeed, the FDA ruling required that any fecal transplant undergo the same scrutiny as a new drug. In other words, a hospital could not perform the procedure unless it was part of a research study, something beyond the capability of most hospitals. (For additional information see (www.fecaltransplant.org/fda-places-restrictions-on-fecal-transplants/,) Hoping the St. Francis doctors were unaware of this development, I chose to keep my mouth shut for fear that that news would mean no return to Birmingham anytime soon, and no fecal transplant anytime, anywhere.

Thanks to the dedicated and relentless efforts of a good and longtime friend, Janice Lasseter, we eventually learned that UAB (the University of Alabama in Birmingham) Medical Center, under the auspices of Dr. Martin Rodriguez, an Infectious Disease specialist, could meet the legal requirements for performing the procedure. And we are fortunate to live in a city with a world-renowned research hospital that had the capability of working with the FDA to research new drugs and new procedures. But UAB had to have an available bed, had to agree to accept Ralph as a patient, and had to work with St. Francis to make the transition from one hospital to another possible. Obviously, that was going to be a tall order.

After days of angst, dogged determination, and the help of St. Francis personnel, we learned that UAB had a bed and was prepared to receive Ralph as a fecal transplant patient. While I was sitting on pins and needles, Ralph was still lying—or trying to lie-- on that tube emanating from his rear end, something more accurately called a bowel management system. We were both fearful that good luck might not hold, that insurance would not cover a new hospitalization, that some unforeseen impediment would impose itself on our plans to leave. On the day of departure, May 16, we experienced any number of delays—the paperwork had not yet been properly completed, the person at UAB who could make the final authorization could not be reached by phone, a 3-hour dialysis had to be completed before Ralph could be dismissed—all these factors fractured our confidence that homecoming was about to be a reality.

At last the hour arrived. I had already checked out of Comfort Suites and said goodbye to the staff there. I had my belongings stuffed in the car, and was simply waiting so that I could leave when Ralph's ambulance left. When I saw the narrow, stiff, unyielding ambulance bed, I was troubled. Ralph's pain-in-the-butt remained unrelenting, and I feared for his comfort. But the ambulance driver and his assistant also understood and had worked with St. Francis doctors to assure that Ralph would have a morphine drip for the long, rough trip to Birmingham. We finally drove away, glad to be headed home but also happy that Ralph had had the good fortune to be treated at St. Francis. I credit that hospital's dedicated doctors, nurses, and staff with saving his life. He still, however, was beset by an uncontrollable *Clostridium difficile* infection.

RALPH:

During my Monroe hospitalization, lying in bed was getting to be agony; I couldn't get comfortable, and, frankly, my butt was very sore. I pushed my call button frequently to ask to be re-situated in the bed—from lying slightly tilted to the left to lying slightly tilted to the right, and vice-versa. I'm sure I tried the patience of the nurses. Sometimes while helping me they would move the call button out of the way and inadvertently forget to replace it where I could reach it. Unable to reach my call button, I would cry for help, and when that happened it often took a long time before anyone heard me. Once when I'd been yelling for help, a nurse came into the room, and I could tell she was annoyed. "Don't be yelling," she admonished me; but her demeanor changed when she saw that I couldn't locate my call button. Misplacement of the call button also meant I couldn't change the TV channel if I wanted to try watching something else, because the call button and the television control were the same device. All those who attended to me agreed that the bed wasn't comfortable and shrugged that there wasn't much they could do. At one point, not long before the end of my stay in Monroe, they actually brought a different bed for me. It was only a slight improvement, but I appreciated their effort. Finally, Glenda went shopping and brought back a soft mattress to put under me. This mattress really made a difference. I felt better about everything then, especially when I knew that soon I might be going home to Birmingham. I even downed some of that awful chocolate protein shake stuff.

When I learned that my hospitalization in Monroe could end with a transfer by ambulance to Birmingham, my spirits rose significantly, not because of anything negative to do with my doctors and nurses in Monroe, but because Birmingham is home. I had always heard good things about the UAB Hospital, and it comforted me and made me more optimistic to know I might be going there. My life had been saved in Monroe, but despite the enema treatments and careful attentions of the doctors and nurses, I was not improving much. Physical and occupational therapists came by my room in Monroe and urged me to let them help me get out of bed and sit for awhile, doing such exercises as alternately raising and lowering each leg. Because of the waste disposal device, I found sitting extremely uncomfortable. Nonetheless, with assistance, I benefited from sitting on the side of the bed and pushing myself up to stand. One Monroe nurse in particular was firm but sweet in her manner of coaxing me to try to get up and sit. She explained what I could see happening: the longer I merely lay in that bed, the more my muscles and strength atrophied. I was weak, and because I wasn't eating anything substantial (was, in fact, still on a jello and broth kind of regimen), I was getting weaker.

27 Days in UAB Hospital

RALPH:

I had my last dialysis session in Monroe the morning of the day I left for Birmingham, May 16. I was excited, anticipating the journey, and more hopeful than I'd been in several days. Time always seemed to drag in the hospital, but this particular day it dragged even more. Finally, around 5 p.m., I was taken from my room to another room where two EMTs awaited. The doctor who originally called Glenda on the day of my hospitalization presided, and he and I signed the necessary paperwork for my departure. The EMTs told me that the ride would be long (a bit over 350 miles) and uncomfortable because I would be lying on what amounted to a hard and narrow shelf in the back of the ambulance. They set up a morphine drip to take the rough edges off the journey for me. I was entirely agreeable to that idea, and I'm sure it helped.

We pulled out of the hospital emergency area and I could see what seemed to me a confusing welter of one-way streets and corners, all near the elevated I-20 where it tracks across downtown Monroe. Soon we were on that elevated Interstate, and I could see the road and Monroe disappearing behind me. I knew the way home from there, having driven it many times, but seeing the highway stretching out *behind* me, often bordered by the flat land of the Louisiana delta, was a perspective I'd never had before. The drone of the ambulance and the hardness of my "shelf" began to coalesce; there was too much noise for conversation with the EMT who was riding along in the back with me, monitoring me as the miles melted away. I dozed, but knew when we were crossing the big bridge over the Mississippi River into Vicksburg; a bit later I knew we were passing through Jackson. I became less aware of where we were as darkness set in, both outside and within my mind. The morphine was doing its work. Once we stopped and got gas. A bit later we came to the site of an accident, where all eastbound I-20 traffic came to a halt. We had to wait quite awhile before we were able to move on. I figured we were getting pretty close to Birmingham, and we were—but it was nearing midnight, and though the EMTs had delivered patients to UAB Hospital before, they had trouble finding the emergency entrance. (We all found out later that the emergency entrance had been moved, so it wasn't where it had been the last time my EMTs had brought a patient to UAB.)

GLENDA:

I had decided I would not try to follow the ambulance back to Birmingham; I would get there on my own. I was instructed to report to the UAB Emergency Room where the ambulance would meet me. Because I was unfamiliar with the exact location of the Emergency Room at UAB, I typed in the address in my GPS and began my trek, stopping along the way for an iced tea and bathroom break and also stopping, against my wishes, several times for extensive road construction. The ambulance, of course, was hampered by the same difficulties. We had not left St. Francis until late afternoon, and so it was well past dark as I approached Birmingham. As I was nearing my destination, I encountered a multi-vehicle wreck that had just happened on the interstate. Traffic had slowed, and people had gathered at the scene. No emergency vehicles had yet arrived, and I was able to go around the crash site and continue on my way. I turned up the volume on my GPS for final directions to the Emergency Room. The outside darkness was unbroken except for some street lamps, and I listened carefully to the GPS instructions, parking on the street when the trusted voice announced that I had "reached my destination." No such luck. I was parked just outside a Wells Fargo Bank branch—in the vicinity of UAB, to be sure, but with no emergency room entrance in sight. And so I found myself circling blocks in the area and finally parking in a place where I could safely leave the car. Once on foot, I could better read signs and locate the emergency room entrance. Thank goodness, I thought, when I finally spotted it not far from where I parked.

Feeling sweet relief, I entered the emergency room, identified myself to the receptionist, gave my husband's name, and told him that Ralph already had a bed assigned to him. Uh-oh. The receptionist had no such record. But after he made some phone calls, he pointed me toward a "no public entryway" route to the hospital proper, to a certain room on the eighth floor. UAB, to a neophyte like me, was a huge maze of hallways, elevators, and medical personnel. With help from the latter, I found my way to the eighth floor and to the room that had been assigned. I cracked open the door and a patient was in the bed. Not Ralph. I returned to the nurse's station, and was told that, "No, your Ralph is not a patient of ours." Nonetheless, they sensed my frustration and discovered by means of computer records that Ralph had, indeed, been assigned a room, but on the *ninth* floor. I returned to the maze, less confusing this time, and found the nurse's station for that unit. Ralph's name was on the list. A very kind nurse told me he had not yet arrived, walked me to his assigned room, and sat with me for quite some time while we waited for the ambulance. Not far behind me in the approach to Birmingham, the ambulance had not been slowed by the accident on the interstate; rather, it had been *stopped* because emergency vehicles attending the crash had by that time arrived and blocked traffic. Because I did not know the reason, I was anxious about the long delay of the ambulance's arrival and about my cell phone's weak signal that wouldn't allow me communication with the ambulance personnel. Because of those stresses, or perhaps because of her understanding nature, I found the nurse's presence and light conversation to be extraordinarily comforting.

RALPH:

Finally, we were at the emergency entrance of UAB Hospital. My EMTs brought me in, and there seemed to be little delay before I was getting situated in a room. Glenda was there, where she had been waiting, she said, for some time. She had driven to Birmingham well ahead of the ambulance, having gotten past the accident site before the traffic jam, and found the emergency entrance with some difficulty. It's hard to express how good I felt to be in Birmingham, where I had every reason to expect continued excellent care and, most of all, could anticipate the fecal transplant procedure that would give me what I now believed would be my best chance to recover. I took considerable comfort in knowing that no one was going to cut away at my colon without first trying the fecal transplant. I knew also that being in Birmingham was a boon for dear Glenda, the end of her 20-day exile in Monroe. Now she could go to our home, sleep in our own bed, and still come to see me each day. We were back in the vicinity of relatives, friends and neighbors, some of whom would come to see me at the hospital.

GLENDA:

I didn't linger long once Ralph arrived and was transferred to his UAB bed. Still bewildered by the labyrinthine hallways, I accepted with relief the kind nurse's offer to escort me down elevators and through hallways; finally, we retraced my steps through the non-public thoroughfare. I thanked my escort nurse, walked outside, located the car, and headed home on familiar roads. Elated to be home but very tired, I washed my face, threw on my pajamas, and crawled into bed—appreciating all the while that it was *my very own bed*. Although it was well past midnight, I couldn't sleep; it took both time and a complaining stomach for me to realize the reason: I was very hungry. Pat, my next-door neighbor, had anticipated my arrival home, and had stocked my refrigerator with some tempting food items. I dished some potato salad onto a small plate and added some potato chips, a rather starchy but tasty combination, I discovered, and downed the both of them with pleasure. I brushed my teeth, crawled again into bed, and fell promptly to sleep.

What a difference good sleep, familiar roads, and daylight can make. The next morning, a Friday, I had little difficulty in locating Ralph's room. I already knew the regimen for keeping germs at bay. Before entering Ralph's room, I donned the gown and gloves that help prevent the spread of communicable diseases. And, of course, those garments had to be disposed of anytime I left the room. Hand washing was critical. Those hand-sanitizer dispensers located beside elevators in hospitals are not equal to the task of killing C. diff. Soap and water are a better answer, as we were reminded time and again by hospital literature. I opened the door to Ralph's room and was pleased to see him in a Birmingham bed, but I was even more gratified to see that nurses had removed the bowel management system—what I had been calling his tailpipe. Nurses—God bless them—were willing to change his diaper as often as necessary. And "often" is an understatement. Poor Ralph would send forth waste, call for a diaper change, get a clean one, and, oftentimes immediately require another one. Small wonder he was losing weight and strength quickly. One thing was certain: time and medicine were not curbing the diarrhea.

RALPH:

Not long after my arrival at UAB Hospital, I met the doctor who was more or less my presiding physician there. I also met the doctor who would be supervising and administering the fecal transplant. They say that home is where the heart is, and they're right; I would add in this case that home was also where my sore butt was, and one of the first things my new doctors did was remove the waste-disposal device from my rectum, ending its

20-day residence there, and ending one of my greatest, abiding sources of bodily discomfort and pain. I was weak, my legs were swollen to almost twice their normal size, my stomach bulged like a huge watermelon (you could even "thump" it), but the worst pain was in my tail, where the waste-disposal device was lodged to carry away the waste from my persistent diarrhea. The removal of the device meant those caring for me would have many diapers to change, but if they minded, they never let on. Now I could occasionally lie directly on my back, and I rested about as well as I could, given that I was still hospitalized and therefore would be frequently awakened by people who needed to check my vital signs, draw blood for tests, change IVs, and so on.

Being free of the waste-disposal device was great, adding to my positive feelings, but another reason I felt so positive occurred when my new doctors, in consultation with a nephrologist, decided to forego dialysis to see if my kidney function would return. In Monroe a great source of relief was learning that as sick as I undoubtedly was, no colon surgery would be required. The Monroe doctor had said I was lucky; I had a fighting chance to save my colon. Now, at UAB, my hopes were further buoyed by being told that my kidneys had a fighting chance to recover on their own. When my catheter was removed on May 22, I was told I now needed to be able to urinate in the usual way. If I didn't "go on my own" within 24 hours, the catheter would have to be replaced. At first I was afraid I wouldn't be able to do so, and I was deeply worried about it.

A nurse—how I wish I could remember her name—often encouraged me to pee during her shift. I was numb around my genitals and wasn't sure I could avoid wetting the bed if I *did* manage to pee. My body swelling and my bed covers moreover made it hard to see what I was doing, even if I could manage to feel that I was holding the urinal in the right place. This nurse therefore helped me by holding the urinal during my attempts to pee, watching for signs of success that stubbornly didn't appear. I was drawing ever closer to the expiration of my 24-hour limit. If I didn't pee soon, I would have to have the catheter put back in. With about two hours to spare, the nurse said, "Let's try this again," and held the urinal in place. I couldn't see, and could barely feel what was going on, but I saw her look up at me with a widening, glorious smile. "Here we go!" she exclaimed, and I probably hadn't been that happy and proud to pee since my toilet-training days. Glenda came in the next morning, and the first thing I told her was "I peed!" She had been worrying the night before about that very thing, trying to think of ways she could help me pee. We were both very happy that morning of Thursday, May 23, but meanwhile, the C. diff diarrhea continued.

GLENDA:

Ralph's kidney function was an issue I worried about daily. His abdomen and legs had been badly swollen the entire duration of his illness, due in part to his kidney failure. Something had to happen, and we were hopeful that he wouldn't have to undergo dialysis treatments the rest of his life. It had been 26 days since Ralph had been able to urinate on his own. When I went home the night of May 22, I slept fitfully, thinking about this crisis, seeing his edema, and trying to imagine ways that I could help Ralph urinate. I wondered if pouring warm water over his genitals would help. I awoke the next morning determined to try something, anything, to make magic happen. When I arrived at his hospital room door, I put on the requisite gown and gloves, entered his darkened room, and heard him proudly announce: "I peed! Three times!"

RALPH:

It was a great feeling to be able to pee on my own, but it's hard to describe how disheartening C. diff diarrhea can be. I got to where I was very reluctant to eat or drink anything because I figured it would just go right through me and make another mess. Often, while aides were cleaning me up and getting me ready for a new diaper, I would feel a rumble in my guts, pass gas, and defecate yet again. I felt embarrassed because I was so utterly unable to help myself. I wanted to apologize, though nurses assured me that there was no reason to do so. At this point I was glad that I still had my colon, glad that I didn't need dialysis, glad to be in Birmingham, but nagged by the inescapable fact that I still had such frequent diarrhea. How frequent was it? Well, months after my recovery, when looking through Glenda's notes for this book, I saw a notation that on Sunday, May 19th, I had 13 stools within a 24-hour period. Such constant diarrhea meant that I was in no way out of the deep woods yet. Glenda and I both pegged our greatest hopes on the fecal transplant, waiting for all the necessary paperwork and permissions to be completed.

GLENDA:

We began making plans with doctors for the fecal transplant, although complications remained. The most notable impediment was the complex paperwork that would convincingly establish the need for the transplant, and subsequently secure the necessary permissions. Behind the scenes, UAB doctors were working with the FDA to get clearance, and we were trying to complete our assignments. We were required to BYOB; that is, "bring your own blender" (a phrase borrowed from someone else who underwent a transplant), along with some coffee filters. I hastened to a nearby discount store and looked at several blenders. Finally, I spotted a Hamilton Beach Wave Station Express, one that promised to "continuously pull mixture down into the blades for smooth results every time." That sounded about right to me, so the purchase was made.

Besides the blender, a donor needed to be identified, preferably someone who either lived in the same home as the patient or someone who had had close contact with him. The donor also needed to be readily available and willing to collect and contribute personal excrement, and provide same-day delivery service. After volunteering, I must have been about as anxious as a beauty pageant contestant awaiting results, but I soon found out that I was a winner—maybe. I had to first prove worthy by producing, *on demand*, a sample to be checked in the lab for evidence that I was clear of such problems as hepatitis (A, B, or C), the HIV virus, syphilis, and *H pylori*. The nurse brought to Ralph's room a neat little kit, including what she called a toilet hat and a specimen cup, for my use. I asked if I was to bring my stool sample the next day. She said, "Oh, no, Sweetie, we need it now." Yuck! This on-demand part was the most difficult aspect of the project, but I went to the hospital bathroom with the supplies provided, placed the toilet hat (and, yes, it looked like a hat) onto the toilet seat, performed my little miracle, then spooned the specimen from the hat into the plastic cup. After turning over my specimen to the lab, I was more than a little pleased to learn the next day that my stool had been sanctioned.

The presiding doctor told us on Friday, May 24 that Ralph had FDA approval for the transplant, and described how the procedure would be done and when. Because Memorial Day was on Monday, the 27th, the transplant was scheduled for Tuesday, the 28th, a date we deemed a promise of relief. Meantime, however, that bright hope was diminished when Ralph developed a urinary tract infection requiring, you guessed it, an antibiotic. The decision was made to do the transplant anyway, as scheduled.

Thus, on Monday evening, I deliberated over what and how much I should eat, what would guarantee that my specimen would be healthy, sufficient, and available for on-time, same-day delivery. Although I had begun taking probiotics, I don't recall what I ate for dinner, but I do know that, despite my tension, I was able to produce the next morning and make the delivery to UAB on time. I was met in Ralph's room by a young pre-med student who accompanied me to the lab where the lab technician received my specimen, the Hamilton blender, and the coffee filters. There, in her lab, she would blend saline and feces until she prepared a solution of the correct consistency (a solution sometimes referred to as slurry), and strain it through the coffee filters. She assured me that the blender would then be destroyed. I didn't stay to watch her wizardry, but returned to Ralph's room where the two of us waited anxiously for the transplant crew and the slurry to arrive.

When they arrived, I was astonished that I was allowed to remain in the room. I sat in a chair, looking and listening as the doctor gave instructions to Ralph while explaining to his medical students this procedure. They were there to learn how fecal transplants might work, a procedure and results they were apparently unfamiliar with. After layering the bed with several pads and towels to catch any leakage, the teaching doctor began by first lubricating Ralph's rectal area, then, while I watched with fascination and trepidation, he inserted the enema nozzle into the anus, slowly and carefully discharged the enema bag contents into the colon, and directed Ralph to hold the solution as long as possible, as much as 30 minutes if he could manage to do so. He and his team then left Ralph with instructions to summon the nurse when he felt he couldn't hold it in any longer. All that went well. Ralph held on for about 30 minutes as directed, the nurses came when summoned, and we began our long wait to see what the results would be.

RALPH:

The day of the fecal transplant, May 28, finally arrived. I had been at UAB eleven days, and it seemed that there were many delays—getting me ready involved paperwork to get approval from the FDA because fecal transplants were considered experimental, and I had a slight urinary tract infection that had to be treated with antibiotics. After the paperwork was finally completed, the transplanting physician decided to go forward with the transplant despite the infection and the antibiotics, but the Memorial Day holiday weekend also contributed to the delays. Glenda had to be identified as a suitable stool donor, which meant that her stool had to be tested. I was eager to get on with it, for I was tired of my daily routines of diaper changes, IVs, taking medications, getting heparin shots in my stomach, frequently holding plastic devices over my nose for what were called "breathing treatments," and occasional visits by occupational and physical therapists who were helping me to sit up and try walking a bit, all with their close assistance. I had a wrist band that indicated I was at risk of falling; I definitely needed their help. Each day I wore very tight support stockings that came up to my thighs, compressing my swollen legs. I saw the fecal transplant as the key to eventually escaping all that. When Glenda's stool was tested and proclaimed free of C. diff and suitable for the transplant, we were both cheered.

On the morning of May 28th, Glenda brought her stool sample to the hospital, along with a brand new food blender for preparing her stool for the transplant. Meanwhile, the transplanting doctor and his team made their preparations for the transplant. UAB is a teaching hospital, so my doctors were often accompanied by several medical students, some of whom assisted with procedures, including this fecal transplant. The acolytes seemed to me to be not only attentive in order to learn, but also genuinely concerned and hopeful for me. The doctor administered the transplant as I lay on my left side. He told me I needed to hold the slurry as best I could for at least 30 minutes, and he made careful note of the time when the procedure was completed. With considerable effort, I held the transplant as directed, aided by my determination and conviction that this, at last, was going to put an end to my ordeal.

GLENDA:

We didn't get the immediate gratification we wanted. We had been told that some patients get results within 24 hours, but that the average time to see positive results was 4 to 5 days. We waited in vain. Ralph never had a solid bowel movement during all this time at UAB, although the diarrhea incidents became less frequent following the transplant. And Ralph did begin to grow stronger. Physical therapists broke through his resistance to sitting up, an activity that at first seemed beyond his capability given his weakened condition. A few minutes of sitting several times a day, a few steps around his bed, an attitude of determination coupled with excellent therapists, finally made it possible for Ralph to leave the hospital unit on May 9, and be assigned to the Spain Rehabilitation Center, part of the UAB complex.

RALPH:

I wish I could report that the fecal transplant was immediately and miraculously effective. We had heard that in some cases C. diff sufferers had improved quickly after receiving fecal transplants, so we hoped for such a result. No such luck. Still, there were encouraging signs, chief among them being that the diarrhea became less frequent. I still didn't like the protein shakes left for me to eat, but my appetite improved. I had some terrific nurses there, and I wish I could remember all of their names. One in particular looms large in my memory. I had been pushing my call button frequently, asking for help in moving around in my bed. The waste-management device had been removed, but I had developed a sore just above where the device had been lodged, and I had trouble staying comfortable enough to sleep. Gently, diplomatically, this nurse told me that I'd been pushing the call button more than I needed to; I needed to make peace with the idea that I just wasn't going to be able to be as consistently comfortable as I'd like. She and other nurses put topical medicine on my sore to help it heal, and they were all good at responding to my various requests, which I tried to limit after my conversation with the diplomatic nurse.

Not long after the fecal transplant, occupational and physical therapists came to my room more frequently than before. Like their predecessors in Monroe, they urged me to flex my legs repetitively while I lay in bed, and move my feet up and down. They pushed me to get out of bed—with their assistance, of course—and sit in a chair for increasingly long periods of time.

They brought a walker to my room and helped me use it at first just to walk around at the foot of my bed; then, later, to walk out into the hallway, increasing my distance from day to day. The firm patience of these therapists cannot be over-emphasized. They were helping me fight off the atrophy of my muscles, the sluggishness of my still-swollen legs, and the lethargy caused by so many days lying in a hospital bed. Doctors also approved more solid food for me, and instead of protein shakes I was brought a product called a "tissue-building powder," a blend of amino acids and carbohydrates that could be mixed with water and tasted much, much better. I knew I was getting better, even though, as seemingly always, I still had bouts of diarrhea. Despite the diarrhea, my doctors thought that soon I could be transferred to UAB's specialized Spain Rehabilitation Center, where I could begin the physical therapy that would eventually enable me to return home at last. After I had been at UAB for 14 days, I was moved to a pleasant, more spacious room in the Spain Rehabilitation Center on Friday, May 31.

GLENDA:

Ralph's room in the Spain Rehab Unit was large, sunny, and cheerful. He learned that he would be required to leave his room twice each day for physical therapy. He was still wearing diapers, having unexpected and unpleasant discharges, but he nonetheless managed to meet the therapy requirements. At times, he would have to stop the exercises to make a quick bathroom trip, but an understanding staff helped him through the difficulties. From May 31 to June 12, he continued his therapy, learning to rise from the bed, lift himself off the toilet, navigate his wheelchair, and, later, his walker. As his strength and capabilities grew, we discussed the transition from hospital to home and tried to anticipate difficulties he might have. Because he had finally advanced to the walker, we opted to leave the wheelchair behind and strive for greater independence once we got home.

RALPH:

UAB's Spain Rehabilitation Center is a splendid, state-of-the-art operation, and soon I became acclimated to their daily routine of rigorous morning and afternoon therapy sessions. It was a new month and I had a positive sense of progress as I was issued a wheelchair, and could soon move skillfully around my room in it, often going to the large windows overlooking the street below. I loved the sunshine that came into the room, and I liked looking at the people and cars moving on the street. I no longer had to take my meals in bed; I could sit in my wheelchair and adjust the table that held my food tray to the desired level. Eager to help me restore strength, Glenda brought me a jar of chunky peanut butter and a spoon from home, so that I could increase my protein intake. I could wheel myself to the bathroom door and, with the help of a therapist, go to the bathroom, then get back into my wheelchair and go to the lavatory to wash my hands, where I could also brush my teeth and shave. Mornings after breakfast, a therapist would come and wheel me to the elevator and then, on another floor, wheel me down to the large therapy area, where I would do various exercises to improve balance and flexibility, and regain strength. I remember working often with an affable and resourceful therapist who had me doing

various tasks, such as stepping up and down on a low stair-step,

raising and lowering my legs, lowering myself onto a bed-level

surface, squeezing rubber balls, playing "catch" with larger balls,

and taking increasingly longer walks up and down the hallways

with my walker. Sometimes I would have some diarrhea

occurrences during therapy, but I was always given assistance to

get to the toilet and, if necessary, get a new diaper. The therapy

continued each morning and afternoon, and I was often quite tired

when I returned to my room. As I improved, therapists helped me

use the shower in my bathroom, showing me how to use the grab

bars and sturdy seat while I plied the soft soap and held the

shower head and directed the flow of the water. They helped me

dry myself off, get dressed, and get back into my wheelchair.

The Spain Rehab supervising doctor visited regularly.

Noting that I was reading a book about the gangster Lucky

Luciano, he surprised me by making comments that proved he

knew quite a bit about Luciano. "They called him 'Lucky,' " the

doctor told me, "because once he was severely beaten and left to die in a swamp, but he dragged himself out, got help, and recovered." I couldn't help daring to hope that I, too, could be "Lucky" and recover; there were frequent signs that I was on course to do just that—but it seemed to be taking so very long, and there was still diarrhea. Occasionally my stool would be semi-firm, and that always gave me hope, but more often than not it was more of a watery mucus-like discharge. Nurses at Spain Rehab were just as good and supportive as my earlier nurses; they changed my diapers and occasionally still held the urinal for me when I was in bed after my evening bath and too tired to ask for assistance in getting out of bed and getting to the bathroom. The supervising doctor was unhappy when he learned that I was sometimes still asking a nurse to bring me the urinal. "That's not rehab," he said, matter-of-factly, and he was doubtless right. Doing more and more for myself—my constant goal in rehabilitation, and as my days in Spain Rehabilitation Center passed and I continued to improve, a social worker visited and consulted with Glenda and me about home-health support services. There were two such services near our home in suburban Birmingham's Hoover area, and when, on June 12, after 12 days at Spain and 27 overall days at UAB, I was released by the supervising doctor to at last go home, we selected one of these services with which to work.

Interlude at Home

GLENDA

June 12 was a huge homecoming day, one I was happy to see although I realized we might have rough sailing ahead, especially so because the diarrhea, although no longer "raging, "remained a daily reality. We had bought some diapers; we had arranged for home nurses and therapists to stop by several times a week; we had food provided by good neighbors (the Conrads, Edmistons, Moxleys, Odoms, Larkins, and Prices), and we were home: all very good things. After getting Ralph settled, I walked onto the patio and discovered, with gratitude and pleasure, that Bill and Vicki Odom had weeded all the flower beds. What a gift! Later, retiring for the night, Ralph and I together in our bed after 47 days of hospitalization, we felt grateful for how far we had come, although the miracle we had hoped for had not happened to the degree we wanted. As we said our good nights, I reminded Ralph to wake me when he had to go to the bathroom.

He did. But not in the way I had expected. He was supposed to reach across the bed and wake me before he tried to get up. Instead, late into the night, he felt the bathroom urge, arose, and was walking around the bed to get me when he fell. The noise woke me, of course, and I said, "Ralph, what have you done?" He was absolutely prone, and had not yet developed the strength to push himself up. No way could I lift him. And so I did what I had been advised by a friend to do: call the fire department. The Hoover Fire Department responded immediately. I unlocked the door, let them in, and by the time we reached the bedroom door, I realized that Ralph had soiled himself. The firemen waited courteously outside the bedroom while I did a hasty cleanup job, then they lifted him carefully into the bed and departed. Anyone who thinks we need to cut government services down to bare bones needs to consider what these dedicated and heroic persons do for us.

RALPH:

It's hard to express the joy and anticipation I felt when Glenda drove me home on Wednesday, June 12. I was back in our neighborhood, back in our home, for the first time since leaving there on April 18, which seemed so very long ago. I was not yet well, but after a total of 47 days, I no longer required hospitalization, and I knew Glenda would continue the excellent care I had prior to my homecoming. The very first night at home, as she helped me get ready for bed, Glenda said, "When you have to go to the bathroom, nudge and awaken me, so I can get up and help you. *Don't* try to go to the bathroom yourself." I hadn't been asleep very long when I awoke and knew I needed to go to the bathroom. I knew I could get out of the bed on my own steam, and so rather than nudging Glenda while I was still in the bed, I got out of bed and began to make my way around the foot of the bed, headed for Glenda's side, where I would then awaken her. That was a mistake. I wobbled as I turned the last corner on her side of the bed, and down to the floor I fell. I wasn't hurt, but I wasn't able to pull myself back up. By now, Glenda was awake, out of bed, and trying valiantly to help lift me up. Despite our best efforts, I could not get up. In my mind I remembered my Spain therapist saying, "Do you know what makes most people fall after they get home? *Overconfidence*. They think they can do something, so they try it and down they go." I was guilty as charged, and to add to my sheepish feeling of culpability, I knew I'd soiled my diaper. The fire fighters came so quickly that they had to wait while Glenda helped me get on a fresh diaper. They helped me up, and I got back into the bed, resolving that I wouldn't try being so prematurely self-reliant again, and I didn't.

GLENDA:

The thirteen days we were home following Ralph's dismissal from UAB are mostly a blur. I remember diapers—lots of them. We developed an almost ritualistic approach for making it through the many diaper changes. Still unable to bend over to adjust his own clothes, Ralph needed my help. Once he had called for me, I would grab a plastic grocery bag, don disposable rubber gloves, get a clean diaper, move his walker out of the way, help pull off the used diaper, and wait just outside the bathroom door until Ralph declared himself ready for additional help. I would then sit on the bathroom floor while I helped Ralph pull up the elasticized clean diaper. We had learned early on that this type of diaper provided not only the best protection but also proved the easiest to maneuver. I would take the soiled diaper (sometimes barely, sometimes heavily soiled), and inspect it in the hope that I would see solid feces instead of the mucus-like discharge that inevitably characterized his output. We had invested so much confidence in the fecal transplant that we had a hard time believing that definite, positive results were not forthcoming. Not once during this time did he have a solid stool.

Unlike his earlier hospital experiences with the C. diff, Ralph now usually knew that nature was calling in time for him to reach the bathroom. There were exceptions: the time in the midst of his shower he felt feces spilling onto the shower floor; the time after showering when he was standing on the bathroom rug when the uncontrollable diarrhea struck, and I asked him to move to the tiled surface to make cleanup easier; the time feces ran down his leg, soiling the bedroom carpet. I scrubbed the

carpet stain with Octagon soap and steamed it as best I could.

Any spills on tile were much easier, and I depended on Clorox—

lots of it—to destroy the spores that made us fear re-contagion.

Soap and water and lots of bleach were part of every routine.

When accidents happened, I resorted to an occasional "Oh, s—t,"

that described what I saw and smelled, but also what I felt. I felt

so sorry for Ralph because I knew he couldn't help these

incidents. What had been happening to him was so

dehumanizing, so distanced from the dignity that differentiates us

from sub-human animals. But it's also true that I felt sorry for

myself. I was also afraid. Optimism was hard to come by when

the dozens of dirty diapers and frequent fecal accidents elicited

fear for our future. We couldn't help but wonder, "How long, oh

Lord, how long can this go on?"

RALPH:

At home, we abandoned the style of diapers that are taped securely at the sides in favor of the style that look like jockey-shorts that can be put on and taken off fairly easily. When I was in the bathroom and needed one of these diapers removed, I still needed Glenda's help, because I was still too stiff and weak to reach down and pull them off without making a mess. Once I had cleaned my bottom, Glenda would start the new diaper by putting it around my ankles, and pulling it up to where I could reach it and finish the task of pulling it into place. I wore these diapers night and day, completing multiple changes every 24 hours. Most of the times that diarrhea struck, the diaper made clean-up and change fairly easy, but inevitably there were times when there was leakage, or some other, more disheartening incident. Such incidents always made me feel bad, not just because they were messy and Glenda had to clean them up, but because I knew they were also proof that I wasn't well yet. Glenda's patience and perseverance through such incidents cannot be overpraised. Hers was a labor of love I can never repay. Through this time, our neighbors were very supportive. They visited briefly on occasion, not wanting to stay too long, but to show their concern. They never failed to offer help if there was anything they could do; some of them gave Glenda a break from cooking by bringing us food.

By now I was taking probiotics (Florastor, Culturelle, Ultimate Flora) and using Cholestyramine for oral suspension—which Glenda mixed with water for me to drink after meals. A home-health care nurse visited two or three times each week, taking my vital signs and answering questions, keeping a close eye on that slowly (but surely) healing sore I had just above my rectum. Occupational therapists visited to make sure I was adjusting to my personal hygiene at home—toilet, shower, gradually doing more dressing of myself. We had a handyman come to install grab bars in our shower and by the toilets in our two bathrooms. Physical therapists visited to suggest strength and muscle-building exercises like walking with my walker and, later, a cane; climbing and descending first just a few, then a few more, of the steps on our stairway to the rooms on the second level of our home. Each morning and afternoon I would get my walker and make multiple trips from one end of the house to the other, passing from our downstairs study through our bedroom, down our hallway past the foyer and living room, past the dining room, and into the kitchen to the door of the garage; then turning and retracing my route.

One of my therapists showed me exercises I could do while bracing myself with both hands on our waist-high kitchen counter, such as rising up and down on my toes; alternating lifting my left and right knees as high as I could; holding first my right, then my left foot lifted straight out several degrees to each side. In our living room she had me repeat sitting and standing exercises in one of our easy chairs; various stretching exercises with stretchable strips color-coded according to their relative elasticity; and repetitive feet, leg, and arm movements. I felt there was little question that I was getting stronger and closer to my abilities before the C. diff struck, though my legs and abdomen were still somewhat swollen.

The diarrhea, however, never seemed to completely go

away, though certainly there were fewer instances of it. On Monday, May 17 we had an office appointment with the infectious disease specialist who had supervised processing the welter of paperwork necessary for FDA approval of my fecal transplant. A sample of my stool was tested for C. diff, and the next day the doctor called us to report that, blessedly, there were no signs of C. diff in my stool. This was great news, and we were further encouraged by our perception that gradually my stool seemed to be getting a bit less watery, another positive sign of recovery. I was, however, still weak, and still needed lots of assistance from Glenda. I continued taking probiotics, and Glenda provided meals that she knew would help restore strength. The home-health nurse and physical therapists continued their visits, and I did my daily exercises diligently. Everything had been a long, slow, slog, but we felt the direction was positive. Then on Monday, June 24, we had a serious setback.

Oh My God, Not Again

RALPH:

The Monday of June 24 began typically, and I was ready when the physical therapist arrived to lead me through my established exercise routines and add a few more, as she usually did. She was pressing me, and I gave her my fullest efforts. We tackled climbing stairs that day, and she added to the number of leg-lifting repetitions and other strengthening routines. When she left, I felt tired, and wondered if perhaps we'd overdone things. If we did overdo it, I decided it was my fault, because the therapist always stressed that I could discontinue whatever we were doing if I thought it was too much. I was so very eager to keep getting better. At any rate, by the late afternoon I wasn't feeling very good. Glenda took my temperature, and I had a fever of 102. I had no appetite and felt so tired I wanted to lie down rather than eat the light, early dinner Glenda had prepared. Worried, Glenda called the home health nurse, reporting my feelings and fever. The home health nurse didn't hesitate in telling Glenda to call an ambulance. I needed more care than Glenda could give me, and despite our mutual reluctance, Glenda called for the ambulance.

The ambulance arrived with Hoover EMT fire fighters who checked my vital signs and readied me for the gurney journey to the back of the ambulance. I thought, well, if I have to go back to the hospital, at least it will be back to UAB Hospital, where I'd received such good care before. But that wasn't to be. The ambulance driver reported that the UAB emergency room was "backed up" with patients and that, moreover, UAB Hospital had no available beds. I was going to have to go to the emergency room at another local hospital (which here will remain nameless). Once again I found myself in the back of an ambulance, watching the road recede behind where I lay, only this time it wasn't I-20 disappearing behind me; it was my own neighborhood. Once again I was producing a list of medications (changed since my earlier hospitalizations, when doctors seemed constantly to fiddle with what I needed to be taking) for an ambulance attendant who was with me in the back of the vehicle. There are no words that adequately express how crestfallen I felt, knowing that I was headed for hospitalization for the third time with C. diff. All I could hope was that this time it wouldn't be as bad. By the time we arrived at the emergency room of this third hospital, I could feel the pressure of the diarrhea.

GLENDA:

We had arrived home on June 12; on June 24, Ralph seemed weaker; he developed high fever, and I called the nurse and reported his condition. She indicated I should call 911 and get him to an emergency room. I did as directed, and, within minutes, the Hoover Fire Department showed up in the fire truck but accompanied by an ambulance. When they asked which hospital I preferred, I quickly said UAB. I trusted their medical staff for the good care they had given Ralph thus far, and I wanted to return to those familiar faces. One of the firemen called ahead, learned that UAB had no bed available, that the emergency room was overflowing, and that another of Birmingham's hospitals had an emergency room that could receive him. I gave the okay to take him there.

Pat Conrad from next door had come over to see how she might help. When she offered to ride with me to the hospital, I gladly accepted her offer. I watched as the firemen took Ralph out the front door to load him into the ambulance. Because I had some paperwork to gather up and my car to load before leaving, Pat and I were a bit delayed in our departure. Not long after leaving the driveway, we caught up with the fire truck and followed it all the way back to the fire station. We couldn't believe, nor did we wish to own, our embarrassment when we realized Ralph could not possibly be riding in a fire truck. The ambulance had left unseen, and in our haste and nervousness we had followed the truck, instead of the ambulance, down the wrong road. We laughed at ourselves, got on the right road, and caught up with Ralph in the emergency room, Pat and I telling each other we shouldn't share our mistake with the world. (Too late; it is now told.)

We had no reason to hurry. The emergency room there began to fill up quickly; it was a rough night in Birmingham, with loved ones and patients waiting their turn for service. Medical personnel buzzed in and around the room where Ralph was temporarily being held, ordering tests, taking temperature, blood, and blood pressure. In the meantime, when Mother Nature couldn't wait for Ralph to have his own bathroom, a nurse helped Ralph out of his bed and delivered him to the men's room down the hall. Left alone, he had a hard time situating himself on the toilet, then lifting himself from it, almost falling as he did so. Meantime, after we spent several hours of waiting for a permanent room assignment, Pat phoned her husband to pick her up. Once she had left, Ralph and I continued the long vigil of waiting, waiting, waiting. Midnight came, and very early on the morning of June 25, he was at last admitted to a room in the hospital. I kissed him goodnight, got in my car, and drove home.

RALPH:

"Emergency Room" is a phrase that suggests quick attention for seriously ailing patients, and it therefore has connotations of relief. But such quick attention is reserved for patients in cardiac arrest or bleeding profusely from accident injuries and the like. Somebody with high fever and diarrhea, however miserable, is not a priority. Once I was received in the emergency room area, it was around 6 p.m. I was checked by an emergency room doctor and occasionally monitored by a nurse, but mostly I waited. When I asked for bathroom help, I was assisted to my feet and pointed to a nearby men's room, where on my own I struggled to get onto the toilet seat. I couldn't get back on my feet after I finished, and I had to call out for help. After that, when diarrhea struck, an aide changed my diaper as I lay in my ER bed. It was after midnight before I was finally assigned to a regular hospital room bed. I understand that lengthy ER waits are to be expected nowadays; after all, most ERs are crowded, often with uninsured patients, and some reasonable system of priorities for attention must be established. Knowing that fact, however, did not make me feel much better while I waited for attention and a room assignment.

I didn't stay long in the first room to which I was assigned. The day after I arrived, I was given medications which included niacin, an over-the-counter capsule that I had been routinely taking at home as a supplement to my blood pressure prescriptions. However, the niacin I had been taking was called "no flush," because I had once taken regular niacin and had had a very uncomfortable reaction to it. Unfortunately, the niacin the nurse gave me at the hospital was not the no flush variety, and soon after I took it, I had an increasingly intensifying feeling of prickly heat spreading through my body. I felt pains in my chest, and immediately told the nurse about them. Trained to be especially alert to patients reporting chest pains, he summoned a doctor who, I presume, was a cardiologist. The doctor asked me about my symptoms, and I told him that I suspected the niacin. Nonetheless, he got on the phone, and I heard him ordering that I should be taken to a part of the hospital's intensive care unit that is dedicated to heart patients. From what the doctor was saying, I could guess that whoever was at the other end of the line was reluctant to admit me upstairs in the heart patient area. "That's not your call," the doctor bluntly said. "I've got a patient here with chest pains, and we're bringing him up." I'm glad this doctor was firmly looking out for my best interests, but I don't know why he ignored my input about the niacin.

And so I found myself in the heart unit where patients with serious conditions such as open-heart surgery were treated, and the nurse in charge there was clearly not pleased to have a C. diff patient on the premises. Of course, my vital signs were monitored; I had all those patches with wires running from them all over my chest, all part of taking an electrocardiogram that was inconclusive. I didn't help my cause by saying that my niacin reaction symptoms had passed, and I *really* didn't help my cause by requiring periodic diaper changes. "We focus on the heart here," the nurse told me more than once, her implications sharply clear. But I had to stay for awhile for observation, and when the attending doctor decided I was okay, the nurse in charge was happy to see me go. I was off to a regular hospital room.

To say that my new hospital room was small is to be generous with language. It was tiny. With the head of my bed to the wall, there were only a few feet on any of the remaining sides between my bed and a wall. There was a similarly tiny bathroom. The walls were a gloomy, drab deep purple-gray. A window allowed some badly needed, almost therapeutic sunshine. I felt somewhat claustrophobic, and of course I felt bad. The doctor in charge of me now was a gastroenterologist with a pleasant, businesslike manner. He confirmed that my C. diff had returned, and he prescribed treatment with Vancomycin and Flagyl, both given orally. So I had to accept what I had feared: The C. diff had returned (if it had ever really gone away), and I was once again going through frequent diaper changes, getting punctured for blood samples, getting various medicines (including the Vancomycin and Flagyl), and being hooked up to an IV. I had nurses and attendants on various shifts who attended to me; some of them were far more professional and seemingly caring than others.

One attendant, however, always seemed patient and cheerful. When once again I needed a diaper change and felt sorry about it, he said, "That's what I'm here for. This hospital isn't going to run out of diapers, so we can get another one anytime you need one." He never failed to put ointment on the sore that was slowly healing just above my rectum. This particular male nurse seemed saintly compared to one female nurse who complained about changing my diaper. Despite the fact that I was hooked up to IVs and had a band on my wrist identifying me as a fall risk, she said, "Why aren't you going in there?" and pointed to the bathroom. Within a day or two of my being in the hospital, one morning a nurse came into my room with one of those waste-disposal devices such as I had had in Monroe. It was clear that there had been a pow-wow, and the nurses weren't going to change any more of my diapers, at least for awhile. So the device was inserted, and once again I couldn't lie flat on my back; I had to be turned to the left or right, and though I tried to move myself in the bed, I often had to call a nurse to help me get comfortable. Moreover, the healing of the sore on my fanny was slowed.

One evening a nurse unhooked me from my IV and moved it into the bathroom so it would be out of the way, and she could bathe me more easily. When she finished bathing me, she left the room and never reconnected me to the IV. I was too groggy to notice her omission, and therefore was just as surprised as the nurse on the new shift in the morning, who asked me, "Where is your IV?" She seemed alarmed as she retrieved it from the bathroom and hooked me back up. On another occasion, it was time for my pain pill, but it wasn't brought. I pressed my call button and asked for my pill, which, I was assured, was coming. Only it didn't. An hour passed and I called again. Then another hour passed, and again I called. Feeling forlorn and neglected, and more than a little angry, I called Glenda, even though I knew she would be asleep at home. When she answered, I said "I'm sorry, honey, but I just have to tell you this," and I unburdened myself. She said she was sorry, she loved me, and she'd call the hospital immediately to complain. By the time I finally got my pain pill, almost four sleepless hours had gone by. A hospital employee charged with asking patients how everything was going came by more than once, inquiring my opinions about my care, and each time I gave a full report, but I might as well have been talking to the drab walls. "Well, we've been short-handed," said the employee, and I didn't doubt it; there had to be some explanation for how long it took to get the medicines I was supposed to get. I was told I'd get a follow-up satisfaction survey to fill out after I was dismissed from the hospital—but to this day I've never received that survey. I realize that many people can and do complain about hospital care, something so expensive yet often unsatisfactory, so at this point I'll give it a rest for awhile.

This relapse and latest hospitalization convinced us both that another fecal transplant was the best route to recovery. My earlier transplant, for whatever reason, had not "taken" as well as we needed it to. Perhaps it failed because of the urinary tract infection I'd had, which required me to be on antibiotics at the time of the transplant. Perhaps the new bacteria cultures from the transplant were not quite able to re-establish a healthy community of bacteria within my colon. Whatever the reason, Glenda did not hesitate to suggest a fecal transplant to the gastroenterologist in charge of my care.

GLENDA:

When the gastroenterologist mentioned treatment options that included a return to some of the C. diff-specific antibiotics that had been tried before (namely, Vancomycin and Flagyl), I asked if we could, instead, try another fecal transplant. I had read of cases where a second transplant was called for, and since Ralph's recovery, had learned that second transplants can have success rates of 99%. The doctor humored me and agreed, and, fortunately, the FDA had by this time eased their recently-imposed regulations. As luck would have it, Ralph was one patient (doubtless there were others) who had undergone the horrors of C. diff at the very same time the FDA had intervened with its stricter requirements. Indeed, it was in April, 2013 that restrictions were imposed, and it was on June 18, 2013 that these same restrictions were relaxed. The timing of this latest ruling meant that our gastroenterologist could perform the procedure that he could not have done a month earlier.

That afternoon I left the hospital early so that I could buy another blender. I wanted no possible excuses to interfere with the upcoming treatment, and I sensed that our gastroenterologist still preferred trying the antibiotic regimen rather than the transplant. Once the decision was made, however, the doctor opted to administer the transplant as an endoscopy rather than as an enema. Wow! If the yuck factor wasn't evident for the enema Ralph had had at UAB, it certainly activated the imagination when I considered that my stool would be going down Ralph's throat—by means of a tube, of course, but the idea was nonetheless distasteful. We were desperate enough, however, to try almost anything. Although we assumed the first transplant had not enjoyed success because of Ralph's urinary tract infection and the antibiotics he was prescribed for that condition, we welcomed a new approach. I let the doctor know that the blender (a different brand this time in hopes of better luck) had been purchased, and that we would be ready for the next try. Meantime, I had to produce once again on demand for the lab tests to assure that my fecal matter would pass muster.

Fecal transplant number two was scheduled for Friday afternoon, June 28. The doctor had visited Ralph's room on the

27th, saw the blender sitting on the window sill, and told me to "Take that thing back; I'll pick out the watermelon seeds." That evening, as well as the days before, I had been trying to eat carefully, for I wanted nothing to go wrong. Thus, on the morning of the big day I arrived gingerly carrying my specimen. By now I deemed my stuff pretty special, and presented it at the lab, much like a toddler in toilet training wanting applause for a deed well done.

This time, I accompanied Ralph to the gastroenterology lab until time for the procedure, but was assigned to a waiting room once the doctor was ready to do his magic. No voyeurism allowed on this occasion, nor did I want to watch this transplant that seemed especially unsavory. The procedure did not take long, but once Ralph returned to the room, another long wait ensued—a very gloomy wait. His hospital room was tiny, crowded with his bed, a recliner, and, later during the recuperation period, a portable potty. There was no room to move around, no room to escape the grim realities of toilets and sickness and aspects of the human condition that healthy people wish to ignore. This grim environment would be Ralph's home for five more days as we began the wait for successful results.

RALPH:

For my part, I was eager to try another fecal transplant, and I told our gastroenterologist so. I didn't want to linger again in the hospital, waiting, hoping, for the oral doses of Vancomycin and Flagyl to work while I played a kind of roulette with nursing care quality. I was happy to see that the doctor was willing to consider the transplant. During the short time since my first fecal transplant, the FDA had relaxed the restrictions on the procedure, making the paperwork much simpler and easier. The doctor told me that he preferred administering the transplant orally by endoscopy in a top-to-bottom fashion that he thought might be more effective. The transplanted solution would then work its way down through my intestines and perhaps have a better chance to re-establish the needed balance of flora. At UAB, the transplanting physician had administered the transplant as a retention enema, a "bottom up" approach that might not have reached far enough into my intestines for maximum effectiveness.

On Friday, June 28, the doctor administered the second fecal transplant via endoscopy. It was the fourth day of my new hospitalization, and my fever was long gone. I was optimistic that this time the transplant would work, and I was eager to recover enough to go back home. I don't recall whether I was encouraged and aided by physical therapists or nurses, but I began again to do some of the in-bed exercises I'd done in Monroe and at UAB. The waste-disposal device was removed, to my considerable relief, and with help of therapists and nurses I could get out of bed and use a walker to walk out into the hall. A portable potty was brought to my cramped room, and when I felt the need, I could call the nurse and, with assistance, get onto the portable potty. Of course, I couldn't always hold it until the nurse came, so diapers again had to be changed with varying degrees of good will. I was getting better, but one recurring problem was that nurses would have trouble finding a good vein to tap when they needed to draw blood for testing. Finally, something they called a "zip line" was installed, making it possible for them to draw blood easily whenever it was needed. I was grateful for that zip line; it meant that I felt less like a human pin-cushion— though I still had to have those heparin shots in my stomach.

Again, improvement was very gradual, and I couldn't yet say with confidence that the transplant had worked. But I knew I was getting better, despite having a dispute with one nurse who, when I requested a bedpan, insisted that every single time I had diarrhea I should get out of bed and use the portable potty. I told her I just wasn't strong enough to do so, that I felt I was doing my best. I didn't see anything wrong with using the bedpan occasionally rather than summoning the strength to get up with assistance to use the portable potty. She painted a dire picture of my failure to recover if I didn't get moving when my bowel got moving. I didn't let her discourage me, nor did I let her convince me that I was doing something wrong. I felt like I was on the right track to recovery, but I realized with some dread that the 4th of July holiday was approaching, and I knew that the short-staffed hospital would be even more short-staffed. I told Glenda I hoped the doctor would let me return home soon because the prospect of being in the hospital through the 4th of July holiday was grim.

The routine testing continued; I remember that after one blood

test I required something I'd never had before in my life—a blood

transfusion. I longed for escape, but I knew I had to get better if I

wanted to leave.

GLENDA:

We were miserable. Nurses and other caretakers were

hard to find when they were needed, although some notable

exceptions brought welcome relief. A young male nurse

reminded me of the servant in Leo Tolstoy's *The Death of Ivan

Ilyich*. In that novella, the peasant Gerasim is the one bright spot

in Ivan Ilyich's life. Confronting the idea of his own mortality,

Ilyich finds that Gerasim is not squeamish about tending to the

bed pan nor any of the tasks associated with alleviating the

suffering of a dying man. Ralph was no longer as near death as

he had been in Monroe; nonetheless, we found comfort in this

young male nurse. Tolstoy's Gerasim was a romanticized

fictional character, to be sure, but this nurse was a real

embodiment of service. When he entered Ralph's room, he never seemed to notice unpleasantness, nor acted as though anything about fecal matter was taboo. When Ralph rang the buzzer for help with a diaper change, this healthy young man responded promptly, pleasantly, and efficiently. Why, I wonder, do such persons receive minimum wage when they are among the most essential caretakers among the many professionals in a hospital setting?

We remained in the hospital until Wednesday, July 3, 2013. Ralph seemed a long way from being well, but Independence Day was the next day. Neither he nor I wanted to remain in the hospital when the unit would be even more understaffed. The doctor agreed to Ralph's release, and we left that afternoon, headed home without the clear results that we were longing for. In preparation for Ralph's homecoming, I had used chlorine bleach to clean as many household surfaces as I could manage. I had read the warnings, chief among them an article in the *LA Times*, wherein the writer, Monte Morin, describes how the C. diff bug "produces hardy spores that can survive for weeks or months in hostile environments outside the body. If a patient touches a contaminated surface, such as a door knob or remote control, and then touches his mouth before washing his hands, he can ingest the bacterium," and start a gut reaction—the multiplication of bad bacteria that can prompt a full-fledged C. diff infection. (www.articles.latimes.com/ . . . /la-sci-feca-transplant-20130117.)

RALPH:

I became rather obsessed with the idea of going home before the 4th of July. I still had diarrhea, but not as bad. I felt I was improving. The doctor said, "Well, nothing is being done for you here in the hospital that couldn't be done at home," and though I knew that meant the burden of my care would again fall upon Glenda, I took heart at the prospect of liberation from that hospital and my tiny room. "You have some issues, though," Dr. Newman said. "For one, you're still having diarrhea, and I thought by now you might not be experiencing that. For another, you're partly dehydrated and you're malnourished. You need to get some good nutrition, especially protein." He didn't sound

very convinced that I was in good enough condition to go home.

As for me, I dreaded the prospect of remaining in my tiny

hospital room and experiencing the quality of care I was having.

The doctor was aware of my complaints, but I don't know

whether he said anything to anyone about them. All I know is

that on Monday, July 1, I asked Glenda to inquire about hiring

someone to stay in my hospital room with me at night—someone

who could make sure I got my medicine and who assisted me in

getting out of bed and onto the portable potty. Glenda said she'd

find someone, and I took some comfort that night that it would be

the last night I'd have to depend on my call button and persistence

to get help.

The next day, July 2, the doctor, though somewhat

hesitant, told Glenda and me that if my condition didn't get worse,

I could probably go home tomorrow—July 3. I'd never heard

better news in my life, and I think my dear, stalwart Glenda felt

the same way, even though she knew my being home would

return her to her prior role of round-the-clock caregiver. An added bonus was our hiring of someone from a home-health agency to spend my last night in the hospital with me. It seemed a Godsend to have her in my room to help me on and off the portable potty, change my diaper when necessary, help make me comfortable, and help nudge the nurses for delivery of my medicines. By now my diarrhea was less frequent, though when it struck it was insistent and strong enough that I couldn't always get to the portable potty in time. The constant presence of the hired caregiver that night made all aspects of my situation better. It was a rather expensive night, as though I'd stayed at a New York City hotel in the theater district ($248.00), but she was worth every penny, especially when you consider that the hospital room cost $1,977 per night. (As I've often said about the ordeal of my illness and lengthy hospitalizations, thank God for my insurance!)

The morning came with a rush of enthusiasm. Today I was going home again, and I was buoyant. Glenda came prepared to take me home, and together we waited in my little room, eager with anticipation. Morning, however, gave way to lunchtime; then the early hours of the afternoon passed. My impatience was making me cranky. Why was it taking so long for my liberation? Nurses came in for routine checks of my vital signs, and to give me medicines. I felt a twinge of desperation: What if, in one of their routine checks, nurses found something wrong? What if I had a fever, or my blood pressure was suddenly too high or too low? What if I suddenly had constant diarrhea? I had allowed my hopes to get so high that the prospect of staying any longer in the hospital was genuinely depressing. At long last, however, the doctor came and signed the necessary paperwork. I was cleared for discharge. The process still took awhile; I had to wait for an orderly to come with a wheelchair, and Glenda had to bring the car around to the entrance where I'd be waiting. It was after 4 p.m. before I was helped out of the wheelchair at curbside and slid into the passenger side of the front seat of our car. I was so happy to see the sidewalks and landscaping around the hospital, so exhilarated to see the wide expanse of blue sky. Progress toward home was slow because the pre-holiday afternoon traffic was heavy. We crawled along Lakeshore Drive, and though I was somewhat concerned that I might have a diarrhea episode during the lengthy ride, I appreciated the attractive homes and expansive grounds around them as we passed. Once we got onto I-65 headed south, the traffic, though heavy, moved faster. Now I felt calm, positive that I could get home without incident. I murmured a prayer of thanks.

Home For Good

GLENDA:

Throughout the house, I had bleached surface after surface, but remained concerned about upholstery fabrics and other surfaces that wouldn't tolerate bleach. I also developed something of a fetish about washing my hands with soap and water, having been told that alcohol wipes and other handy germ killers—sprays and wipes—were ineffectual against the C. diff spores.

Once we were home, accidents happened, and diapers were still needed. Often when inspecting the diaper, Ralph would report, or I would see for myself, that the discharge was soiled mucus. I was wondering if my transplanted stool had been sufficiently healthy, and I feared that no doctor would opt for a third transplant. Something wonderful, though, was about to happen. UAB's Dr. Rodriguez had already scheduled us for a follow-up visit on July 8, and while we were dressing and preparing for that appointment, Ralph felt the bathroom urge. He went, and produced a solid bowel movement for the very first time since mid April, and a few hours later he did it again to provide a testing sample for Dr. Rodriguez!

RALPH:

Now that I was again home, it was once again time to engage my illness for the long haul of recovery. We re-established connections for home health services such as nurse and physical therapist visitations which began again. I wasn't hospitalized long enough to lose all of the ground I had gained before the relapse. My legs and abdomen were not as badly swollen, and I resumed my repetitive walker-assisted trips through the house. With the therapist I returned to my exercises: "marching," in which I alternately raised each leg as high as I could, up and down; rising onto my tiptoes repeatedly; alternately bending my knees backward, bringing my heels as high as I could; repeating a slight squat; and the like. The therapist also worked with me in stretching in various ways the elastic strips that were color-coded to indicate different levels of stretch resistance. It was a triumphant day when, with the therapist's supervision, I made it all the way up the flight of stairs leading to my study, where before my illness I typically spent long hours writing. As these physical strides unfolded, I resumed, with Glenda's assistance, the most nutritious diet I could. I made sure I had plenty of protein, and I took probiotics. I still had some diarrhea and required Glenda's assistance in bringing me jockey-short style diapers and making sure I didn't fall while getting into and out of the shower, where I sat on a sturdy plastic chair and used a flexible hand-held shower head. Her patience with me was lovingly enduring.

Glenda and I were both highly encouraged when Dr. Rodriguez called to report that my latest stool sample was free of C. diff. That was good news, but of course I couldn't help remembering that my stool had tested free of C. diff before my relapse and re-hospitalization. My optimism was therefore cautious, and it remained so. Some fecal transplant patients have positive results quickly, within three or four days of the procedure. For me, the positive result came about ten days after the transplant, just before my visit to Dr. Rodriguez' office.

Thereafter, subsequent stools at home were normal and showed

no traces of diarrhea. Moreover, I was now having only one or

two bowel movements each day, and I continued my therapy and

required less and less assistance in any way. Without realizing it

as these signs of recovery kicked in, I became more quietly

determined, concentrating so much on recovering that I often fell

silent and unresponsive when Glenda spoke to me.

GLENDA:

Sickness can be insidious. Symptoms of a disease can

cast long shadows across our future, leaving us, its patients and

the patients' companions, to wonder what power this enemy had

to affect our plans for a long and healthy life, to travel, to visit

grandkids, to pursue the upcoming years with relative ease.

There are also shorter shadows, the immediacy of the illness, the

way it crowds out mundane routines and pleasures. We

experienced both kinds of shadows in our pursuit of good health.

We cancelled our annual trip to the Inge Festival in

Independence, Kansas; we had to prepare the paperwork to cancel a European trip we had long planned for; we were no-shows at a family reunion; we were unable to meet friends for dinner; and were we not retired, we would have had to take long leaves of absence from our places of employment.

The shadows you don't talk about can be the most sinister. Illness takes its toll on relationships, even very good ones. All the energy the patient can summon is focused on getting well. The caretaker wants validation as she expends her energy in waiting on the patient, doing the extra laundry and cleaning, responding to inquiries about the patient's health. What happened in our case was a spell of silence. I asked Ralph if he wanted homemade vegetable soup for dinner. Silence. I mentioned that a flower was blooming in the backyard garden. Silence. I asked how he felt. Silence. I couldn't get past my own sense of persecution to understand what was happening to Ralph's will to get well and why I was receiving the silent treatment. When Betsy and Johnny came to visit, they, too, noticed his silence, and began to worry about me.

Because I needed a second driver, I had been postponing getting Ralph's truck cleaned. When Betsy came for another visit, we decided this was a good time to take it to a local detail shop to have it steam cleaned, the best treatment I could imagine for destroying any C. diff spores that remained. I drove the truck; Betsy, with Ralph as her passenger, followed me in the car so that all of us could immediately return home and not have to wait for the truck cleaning to be completed. Once we returned home, Betsy asked me about what was going on. She had tried to make conversation, even asked questions of Ralph, but got only silence for response. I told her that I didn't understand what was happening.

What I did understand was that something had changed. During most of Ralph's sickness and recuperation we had had a sense of "we're in this thing together," but during one phase of the recovery there were a couple of painful weeks when that did not seem to be the case. We were two separate human beings struggling within the shadows we had allowed to fall between us. One morning when a neighbor called, I answered the phone to find a cheerful voice on the other end. Engaged in the conversation, I didn't hear Ralph call to me that he was headed to the bathroom and needed diaper assistance. When I returned to the living room, Ralph confronted me with, "Where were you? I needed a diaper and you weren't there." I broke into tears and defended myself with, "I'm doing the best that I can." In describing this scene, I realize that it focuses on what Ralph did to me—the blame game. The point, however, is that serious illness can make a different person of you, at least for awhile. Ralph, my kind and thoughtful husband, had become so unlike himself; because I didn't know how to cope, I, too, became another person, and was surrendering with feeling-sorry-for myself tears and misplaced anger.

RALPH:

Looking back on it, I'm not sure I can account for my lapse into the silences and occasional flare-ups. I think I was a little depressed because, despite my gradual improvement, that improvement seemed so infinitely slow. I missed my formerly healthy self; I was so tired of being sick, being constantly in recovery mode that, however positive a direction, moved at a glacial pace. I didn't feel very social when Betsy visited, though I knew Glenda was glad to have a supportive and loving alternative to my constant, demanding company. I selfishly thought mostly of myself, my need to continue therapy, continue walking through the house with my walker, doing my exercises, and the like. I just wanted to be back to where I was before I left for Austin the previous April. My progress just seemed to be so slow, and I was drawing into myself much more than I realized, and more than was good for my relationship with Glenda. I realize now that I had started to take her care and attention for granted, and I had stopped responding to her appropriately. When she cried that she was doing her best, I snapped out of it.

GLENDA:

On later reflection, I think much of the tension between us was because of constant togetherness. We had each other, and that was about all. Friends and family were exceptionally kind, but possible contagion made it unwise for them to visit, and, because of the insistent diarrhea, we were unable to go anywhere. We were constant companions both night and day, and our roles as equal partners, as husband and wife, had devolved into patient and caretaker. While Ralph was in Birmingham hospitals, I had the selfishness and/or the wisdom to seek fresh air. At UAB, I would leave the building most days for lunch, walk outside for a few minutes, locate a nearby place to order lunch and sit by myself and meditate. Or on other occasions, my sister Becky or my friend Hilda would meet me for lunch, and I could enjoy their company and the diversion those conversations offered. Likewise, while still in Monroe, I enjoyed pleasant lunches with Ralph's sons—John, Walker, and Collin—whenever they were visiting. At home, though, there was no escape, no metaphoric fresh air entering our sick space and providing relief.

Once I had my tearful outburst, I'm glad to report, tensions were released. The anger and the silence were soon replaced once again with the business of getting well. The tears had prompted healing conversations. When the shadows began to disappear and became part of remote memory, we smiled at each other and managed to talk pleasantly about our everyday lives, even if that talk was about bowel movements that continued to be healthy and regular. Ralph's walker was soon replaced by a cane. The most promising sign of all: I would hear Ralph singing in the shower. We began making local trips by car, and found more opportunities to connect with friends and family. Unlike many in America, we were fortunate to have good insurance, so medical expenses were not a huge issue for us. I couldn't help but think about persons in the same crappy boat who had concerns not only about getting well, but also worries about how in the world they could ever pay the enormous medical bills they were racking up.

RALPH:

After Glenda and I worked through the difficult time of silences and negative feelings, I returned to a more positive demeanor. Being able to discard first my walker and then my cane, I was heartened to be able to climb the stairs to my study in our home. My study is important to my sense of myself; there I read and write to my heart's content; my books and recorded music are nearby, with my collection of movie video cassettes and DVDs. My guitar is on a stand near my desk; I can pick it up and strum chords and sing whenever I wish. As days of therapy passed, I also began to anticipate once again driving. I'd been cautioned throughout my therapy that my auto insurance would be no good unless I'd been released from therapy and approved for driving by the UAB doctor in charge of my physical rehabilitation therapy. The day of my appointment with that doctor arrived, and though he seemed pleased at my ability to pass the tests he gave me, he was not nearly as pleased as I. We left his office and I couldn't wait to get home, get into my truck, and take a short spin in our neighborhood. It was a grand feeling. For Glenda and me, our lives began to settle back into our customary pre-illness routines. As I write this, more than a year later, I dare to hope that the C. diff will not return. All I can say is that so far, it has not. Glenda and I have begun to travel again. We are both deeply thankful.

Going Forward from Here

Ours is a cautionary tale. We were both born in 1943, the same year that a laboratory worker, Mary Hunt, discovered a mold inside a cantaloupe with "a pretty golden look." Following the initial discovery of penicillin by Alexander Fleming in 1928, Hunt, along with other scientists, had been looking for an efficient way to produce sufficient quantities of our first antibiotic, and needed a particular strain that would address this need . The demand for a miracle drug was critical not only to treat illnesses such as pneumonia, but especially to treat World War II soldiers who were losing limbs and dying from uncontrollable infections that developed from their battlefield wounds. Hunt's discovery was timely, for her cantaloupe had the right strain of *penicillium*—one that could be grown in very large fermentation tanks, considerably advancing the development of the drug we know as penicillin, as well as its widespread distribution. Other miracle drugs would soon follow, and our generation would make them part of our medical lives.

(www.herbarium.usu.edu/fungi/FunFacts/penicillin.htm)

Our parents' generation was enthusiastic about penicillin, and it was becoming widely available and frequently used as Glenda was growing up on a small Alabama farm about two miles from the center of her little town, and Ralph was growing up on the edge of his little Kansas town. Mostly we ignored bumps, bruises, and sniffles; we had our teeth pulled or filled without Novacaine, and excepting common childhood diseases of the time, such as measles, chicken pox, and mumps, we were seldom sick enough to miss school for more than a day or two. But if the flu hit, Glenda's dad would say, "Take that girl to the doctor and get a shot of penicillin." We wanted those penicillin shots even if our flu was the result of a viral rather than bacterial infection. The penicillin was there for us if we needed it. Glenda's folks had a barn with mice that they killed with some kind of poison, and they had a back porch with flies that they attacked with an insecticide called "Fly Flakes" (a DDT product). We were both exposed, therefore, to both the good and the bad that the post-war generation had to offer: the miracle drugs to cure us, and the poisons that adversely affected our environment. We've come a long way since then, with DDT no longer accepted, and most of us questioning the kinds of insecticides and poisons we use. But we have glibly and irresponsibly found antibiotics too easy a solution for what ails us. Their indiscriminate use has contributed to an alarming increase in super-bugs such as MRSA and C. diff.

Antibiotics lose their effectiveness as disease-causing bacteria develop resistance to them. We are, therefore, on the threshold of a crisis because common infections once successfully treated with antibiotics are, today, potentially life-threatening. The development of new, more powerful antibiotics has not kept pace with our need to outsmart the resistant bacteria. Indeed, in a 2014 report, the World Health Organization reveals "that it is no longer a prediction for the future. Antibiotic resistance—when bacteria change and antibiotics fail—is happening right now, across the world." These evolved bacteria, having grown resistant to the antibiotics we use, have become known as super-bugs and are a "major concern because a resistant infection may kill, can spread to others, and imposes huge costs to individuals

and society." Even minor injuries and ordinary infections, once

controllable, can now be lethal. (See www.who.int/en/.)

To complicate still further the antibiotic dilemma: those

of us from industrialized nations do not make ideal fecal donors.

According to Alexander Khoruts, gastroenterologist and

immunologist at the University of Minnesota in Minneapolis, the

gut microbiomes of all westerners have been compromised by our

history of antibiotic use. Ideal donors, Khoruts claims, are people

from Africa or the Amazon, whose microbiomes replicate the

diversity of their pre-antibiotic ancestors.

(http:www.bbc.co/future/story/20140429-medicines-dirtiesst-

secret)

Yet another argument against our overuse of antibiotics is

presented by researchers at the University of Alabama in

Birmingham. Dr. Richard Whitley, for example, warns that we

need also to "get antibiotics out of the husbandry food chain." He

is referring to the heavy dependence of agribusiness on

antibiotics, a mainstay of animal husbandry used to maintain animal health, and also to make animals in feed lots—beef, chicken, pork—gain weight quickly. These meat products, in turn, can pass along drug-resistant bacteria to us if we eat undercooked meat, or if we are exposed to bacteria by means of contaminated food preparation surfaces (Courtney Haden, "Triumph of the Bugs," *Weld*, May 8-14, 2014). Awareness of the perils of excessive antibiotic use and C. diff has been rapidly growing. A smattering of Glenda's research has revealed a good deal about this growing awareness.

GLENDA:

I began my own research with my constant companion, my iPad. It turns out that Ralph's experience with this infection coincided with an uptick in public information about the widespread outbreak of C. diff, especially in hospitals and nursing homes. Reporting on a *USA Today* investigation, Peter Eisler observes that C. diff is "linked in hospital records to more than 30,000 deaths a year in the Untied States . . . strik[ing] about a half-million Americans a year." Numbers of deaths vary among the various publications, he reports, due in large part to the fact that death certificates often list a complication (such as kidney failure) as the reason for the death rather than C. diff itself. During the last decade C. diff rates have been rising, while other super-bugs have been on the decrease. In fact, C. diff deaths represent "nearly five times the rate of other hospital stays." (www.usatoday.com/news/health/story/2012-08-16/deadly-bacteria-hospital-infections/57079514/1.)

Those infected with C. diff have usually been on a broad spectrum antibiotic regimen, often for some illness originally unrelated to their C. diff. Indeed, we, the public, have made our friend—modern medicine—our enemy as we have relied too heavily on the use of antibiotics to make us well from all sorts of infections, and these drugs, in turn, have all too often proved themselves enemies to our colon health. Successful treatment of C. diff has therefore become more difficult. Ironically, other antibiotics, very specialized ones such as Vancomycin and Flagyl, have been the usual approach for clearing up C. diff, but they have proved less effective in recurrent and severe cases. Another antibiotic, Dificid, has proved somewhat more effective in attacking C. diff. Dificid, however, is extraordinarily expensive—approximately $3,150.00 for 20 pills at discount pharmacies, and that's with a coupon. As we write this, ongoing research seeks to develop other antibiotics to treat C. diff.

Yet another *USA Today* report, referring to the work of gastroenterologist Josbert Keller, describes how a healthy gut is constituted of beneficial, necessary microbes. In fact, "100 trillion bacteria, fungi, and other microscopic bugs live in and on the human body without which people would not survive." When our healthy gut bacteria are destroyed, along with the bad bacteria that are the target of the antibiotics we take for sickness, we are in trouble. Disappointed in the failure of modern medicine for wiping out C. diff, Keller, who practices medicine in Amsterdam, is among a growing number of physicians who have turned to non-standard treatments; i.e., fecal transplants, and have found them superior to the specialized antibiotics normally used. In his study, two groups were established for comparison purposes. The results: 15 of the 16 fecal transplant patients were cured, whereas only 7 of 26 receiving antibiotic-only therapy were cured. (www.usatoday.com/story/news/ . . .fecal-transplants/837575.) Perhaps no journalist has been more engaged with the potential for fecal transplants for restoring health than has Maryn McKenna. She explains how the transplants work when other procedures fail. What we have with fecal transplants, she says, "is a treatment that is minimally invasive, reliable, cheap, and with a long clinical history," all with a cure rate of 90%.

(www.wired.com/wiredscience/2011/12/fecal-transplants-work/.)

I also learned what the wise animal kingdom has known all along: poop, good poop, is essential for our well being. Elephants, koalas, pandas, and chimpanzees are among those animals who engage is coprophagia, "the consumption of feces." For some, the poop is a source of protein; for others, such as the elephant and koala, the ingestion of poop is necessary for preparing the newborn's sterile digestive tract with the necessary bacteria needed for digestion once the animal begins eating the vegetation that is part of its ecosystem.

(http://en.wikipedia.org/wiki/Coprophagia.) I also heard, by way of the grapevine, that veterinarians as early as the 1950's successfully treated racehorses' diarrhea with fecal enemas. Indeed, my research uncovered much of interest to victims of C. diff and their caretakers.

RALPH AND GLENDA:

We could add much more that we've found out about excessive antibiotic use, C. diff, and its symptoms, treatments, and results. But the picture is clear: C. diff infections are on the rise, and some cases are very serious, life-or-death matters. It's our opinion, one shared by many in the medical community, that antibiotics, especially broad-spectrum antibiotics, should be prescribed sparingly. And it is also our opinion, not yet widely shared in the medical community, that fecal transplants should be the *first* resort in treating recurrent, severe cases of C. diff—not the *last* resort. For more information about the rise in C. diff awareness, research, and treatment, see our list of sources.

Finally, we must say something in general about the costs

of our medical care. They were so high that without our good health insurance—Medicare and Ralph's supplemental insurance via his retirement package—we would have been bankrupted. Wiped out. We don't pretend to know what solution there is, if any, for the many, many uninsured people in our country. But there is no doubt that countless uninsured people go untreated because they cannot pay, or, if they are treated, they have no hope of paying. And that strikes us as tragic in the U.S., where the best medical treatment in the world is possible.

As we write this, we're past the first-year anniversary of Ralph's battle with C. diff. Springtime is happening, with pine tree spores abounding, reminding us of the teeming life forces at work all around us and within our own bodies. We hope this little book can be read not only as a hymn of praise to those wonderful microbiome communities that determine our health, but also a narrative about how fecal transplants, while not the answer for everyone, proved a miracle for us. It has been a difficult year, but one that has challenged us to be more responsible in our use of antibiotics and more appreciative of the wonders of nature. And it has also been the year, as Ralph has noted elsewhere, that "we,

Ralph and Glenda, finally got our s. . .t together."

Glossary of Terms Used in This Book

Antibiotics

Antibiotic medications have become a commonplace approach for treating infections caused by bacteria. Penicillin was our first antibiotic and was hailed as a miracle drug when it became available in the 1940s. It and other modern antibiotics have been overused and are, therefore, creating a public health threat, as harmful bacteria have developed a resistance to antibiotics and have evolved into what are commonly called "super-bugs."

Antibiotic Resistant Super-bugs

Infections that are resistant to antibiotics. Super-bugs are proving themselves superior even to those antibiotics prescribed as "last resort"--due in large part to antibiotic overuse. Super-bugs are currently in the news because they are wreaking more and more havoc in nursing homes, hospitals, and even in private homes. Some noteworthy super-bugs include MRSA, E. Coli, and C. diff. Among these, C. diff is, at present, proving one of the most difficult to treat.

Bowel Management System

Often used in hospitals and nursing homes for incontinent patients who lack mobility. This device is designed to divert feces away from the patient and provides a method of containment.

Broad Spectrum Antibiotics

Antibiotics that attack a wide range of infectious bacteria. Generally used when the source of infection is unknown, or where there are multiple types of bacteria that are causing illness.

Clostridium difficile ("C. diff," for short)

A potentially quite severe illness caused by a bacterium of the same name. Complications of C. diff infections include diarrhea that can cause significant dehydration and consequent loss of fluids and electrolytes, leading to low blood pressure; possible kidney failure, toxic colon; and other serious bowel damage that could prove fatal.

Colonic Flora

Bacteria that live in our digestive tracts, making up part of our microbiome community. We can have both good and bad bacteria; unless we have sufficient quantities of the good flora to hold at bay the bad bacteria, the bad bacteria can take residence in our gut, colonize, and cause problems such as a C. diff takeover. The microbiota in our gut have been called "a complex bacterial consortium that is critical to normal health" (www.jn.nutrition.org/content/134/2/459-full). Health professionals are perceiving our gut flora as far more important than previously thought. Ann M. O'Hara and Fergus Shanahan, for example, describe how this flora "has a collective metabolic activity equal to a virtual organ within an organ." We can expect to see breakthrough developments in the near future as scientists study the importance of this influential "organ."

(www.ncbi.nim.nih.gov/pmc/articles/PMC150832)

Dificid (fidaxomicin)

A narrow spectrum antibiotic that targets C. Diff bacteria with less damage to other intestinal flora than some antibiotics. Currently very expensive.

Fecal Transplants

Often referred to as Fecal Microbiota Transplant, this procedure can involve the use of a donor's fecal matter that is mixed with saline solution and inserted in the C. diff patient's body to colonize the intestine with healthy flora. Delivery can be by colonoscopy, enema, or a nasogastric tube that sends the fecal slurry into the stomach by way of the nasal passage and throat. Sometimes the fecal matter is administered in capsules taken orally, and sometimes the treatment is used to combat Crohn's disease and other disorders of the digestive tract. At this writing, fecal transplants are still widely considered experimental, although current research is demonstrating impressive efficacy.

Flagyl (metronidazole)

An antibiotic prescribed to stop the growth of bacteria and protozoa—often the drug of choice when C. diff infections first occur.

Florastor

A yeast-based probiotic that is taken orally to help build healthy gut flora.

Human Microbiome Project

Published in 2008, the Human Microbiome Project investigated the little-understood population of bacteria that reside in and on our bodies and influence our health. In terms of our particular interest, this research shows promise for demonstrating the role our microbiome community plays in diseases and infections, especially the development of C. diff. This field of study is now wide open for scientific investigation, with possibilities for new approaches to a variety of diseases and disorders. Indeed, never before in medicine has there been such a fascination with our bodies' microbes, especially human stool.

Kidney Dialysis

The dialysis machine assumes the task of filtering the blood and ridding it of waste products, a job healthy kidneys normally do.

Muscular Atrophy

A dissolution of muscle. The loss of muscle mass leads to muscle weakness and the muscles' inability to perform certain tasks, such as walking.

Narrow Spectrum Antibiotics

Antibiotics that have been developed to address a narrow range of microorganisms. Considered less likely than Broad Spectrum Antibiotics to cause C. diff.

Probiotics

Bacterial or yeast organisms that can help restore or maintain a healthful digestive tract, probiotics come in a variety of brands readily available without prescription.

Pseudo Membranous Colitis

An inflammation of the colon often caused by C. diff. Symptoms include diarrhea, fever, and abdominal pain.

Retention Enema

An enema introduced into the rectum and sigmoid colon; the patient is asked to hold the solution for a prescribed amount of time—from a few minutes to an hour or two.

Rhabdomyolysis

A destruction of skeletal muscle tissue that occurs when myoglobin (the protein contained in muscle cells) is excreted in the urine. Rhabdomyolysis can cause muscle pain and weakness, and can prompt kidney failure when the kidneys' filtering system becomes clogged with the myoglobin that has spilled into the blood stream.

Sigmoidoscopy

This procedure provides important knowledge to the physician who uses a flexible endoscope or a rigid device for looking at the inside of the large intestine—up to the sigmoid. A tube with a light is inserted, and an image of the rectum and colon is transmitted, allowing the doctor to discover such things as diarrhea, constipation, internal bleeding, ulcers, inflammation, and unusual growths.

Vancomycin

A drug of choice for many doctors treating C. diff. Oral Vancomycin is not designed for treating infections in other parts of the body, but IV Vancomycin is a commonly used antibiotic for infections such as MRSA.

Acknowledgments

It probably seems ridiculously obvious to express our gratitude to the many doctors, nurses, therapists, and other health care professionals who helped us in so many ways during and after our long battle with C. diff—but we nonetheless do acknowledge them and their expertise and humanity. We shall always be grateful. Among these doctors are, alphabetically, John Bruchhaus, Greer Burkholder, Clayton Coon, Michael Hand, Mark Napoli, Randy Newman, Anthony Pitts, Martin Rodriguez, James Smith, Darlene Traffanstedt, and Nicholas Van Wagoner. Among technicians and nurses we want to thank are Kimberly Beasley and Paula Dixon, and particularly Jennifer Saltzman, the night nurse at UAB Hospital who guided Glenda through the hospital maze and comforted her during the long night while Glenda waited for Ralph to arrive by ambulance to Birmingham from Monroe. We regret not knowing all the last names of these nurses we also want to thank: Jake, Jessica, Kim, and Robin. Spain Rehabilitation Center has many great therapists, and we thank Steve in particular. A home-health nurse, Sonya, spent Ralph's last night in the hospital with him, easing the difficult time he had been having. There are other medical and therapeutic professionals for whom we have no names, but they are Samaritans all, and we are grateful.

We want also to thank Barbara French, whose loss of her husband to C. diff inspired some of our early research into fecal transplants. Barbara and her daughter Molly shared their research with us and played a big role in helping us to begin our road to recovery. We thank members of the "Prayers and Squares" quilting group of the Church of the Resurrection in Loudon, Tennessee, who sent Ralph a colorful prayer quilt on which "each knot represents a prayer that was said" for him. Such sentiments help healing. Seldom do people realize what a difference small gestures mean in making stressful days less so; thus, we owe a huge debt of gratitude to the staff at Comfort Suites in Monroe, especially Janice, Shay, and Sharon, who eased Glenda's stay for 21 long days. And thanks to Hilda Hicks for the phone conversations and care package. We appreciate the ambulance crews in Monroe and Birmingham who transported Ralph to hospitals. Thanks also go to the strangers who expressed kindness and concern to Glenda as she gathered with them in the waiting room at St. Francis Medical Center in Monroe, and to the Hoover, Alabama Fire and Rescue personnel who twice came to our home when Ralph was in trouble. We both have many relatives whose love and concern helped sustain us during the ordeal: Glenda's children, Betsy and Johnny; her sisters Sandra and Becky, her brother Roger; her cousins, and her great-nieces and nephews who sent get-well drawings and made home videos; Ralph's sisters Betty, Joyce, Grace, Shirley, Alice, Marilyn, and their families; his cousins, nieces, and nephews; his sons John, Walker, and Collin; and many others far too numerous to mention who were recipients and responders to Glenda's email bulletins. Our gratitude also goes to friends and neighbors, especially Pat and Jim Conrad, Bill and Vickie Odom, Rob and Lydia Moxley, Tom and Kathy Nequette, Bob and Karen Price, Doug and Lisa Beckham, Willie and Judy Edmiston; Luedean and Jim Larkin, Phil and Rosemary Kimbrell, and Janice and DeWayne Lasseter.

There are so many other good people, also too numerous to name, who showed their unwavering love and support for us during Ralph's long hospitalizations and recovery. Their cards, flowers, notes, favors, visits, meals, and other many kindnesses and thoughtfulness gave us hope, strength, and steadfast reassurance.

Sources and Suggested Readings

Some of our sources are embedded in our text and not listed here; some are both embedded in the text and listed below. The list is not intended to be exhaustive, but it is highly representative of what is available to those who want to know more about C. diff.

ON THE WEB

www.articles.latimes.com/ . . /la-sci-feca-transplant-20130117

http://www.bbc.com/future/story/20140429-medicines-dirtiest-secret

http://cdifffoundation.org/

http://en.wikipedia.org/wiki/Coprophagia#See_also

www.fecaltransplant.org/fda-places-restrictions-on-fecal-transplants/

www.huffingtonpost.com/2012/04/09/c-difficile-fecal-transplant_1413119.html

www.jn.nutrition.org/content/134/2/459-full

www.mayoclinic.org/diseases-conditions/c-difficile/basics/definition/con-20029664

www.ncbi.nim.nih.gov/pmc/articles/PMC150832

www.news.msn.com/science-technology/wonder-cure-for-gut-fda-allows-fecal- transplants

www.nytimes.com/2010/07/13/science/13micro.htm/

www.sciencedaily.com/releases/2007/09/0709051.7450/

www.smithsonianmag.com/science-nature/the-unintended-2nd

www.uab.edu/news/latest/item/2489-defined-healthy-microbiome-to-shake-up- understanding-of-many-diseases

www.usatoday.com/news/health/story/2012-08-16/deadly-bacteria-hospital-infections/57079514/11

www.usatoday.com/story/news/ . . .fecal-transplants/837575

www.who.int/en/

www.wired.com/wiredscience/2013/01/fecal-clinical-trial/

www.wired.com/wiredscience/2013/5/fecal-transplants-fda/

https://www.youtube.com/watch?v=4oA6QgaUdlY (Preview)

www.wired.com/wiredscience/2011/12/fecal-transplants-work/

IN PRINT

Bakken, John S. "Staggered and Tapered Antibiotic Withdrawal with Administration of Kefir for Recurrent Clostridium difficile Infection." *Clinical Infectious Diseases,* September 15, 2014, pp. 858-861.

Belluck, Pam. "A Promising Pill, Not So Hard to Swallow." *New York Times,* October 12, 2014, p. A21.

Butler, Kiera. "Does Your Germophobia Breed Superbugs?" *Mother Jones,* January-February 2014, pp.66-67.

"Dire Infection, One-Day Cure." *Good Housekeeping,* November, 2013, pp.100-103.

Dubberke, Erik M.D., and Curtis Donskey. *Contemporary Diagnosis and Management of the Patient with difficile.* Handbooks in Health Care Company, 2011.

Eakin, Emily. "The Excrement Experiment." *The New Yorker,* December 1, 2014, pp. 64-71.

Haden, Courtney. "Triumph of the Bugs." *Weld.* May 8-14, 2014, no pagination.

Keener, Vicki. *What Is C. Diff, Its Symptoms and Treatment.* 2013. Kindle only.

Laliberte, Richard. "Is Our Drug Habit Killing Us?" *Good Housekeeping,* April, 2014, pp. 75-82.

Lamont, J. Thomas, M.D. *C Diff in 30 Minutes: A guide to Clostridium Difficile for Patients and Families.* i30 Media Corporation, 2013.

Marchione, Marilynn, Pills Made from Poop Go Straight to Gut of Problem." Memphis *Commercial Appeal,* October 4, 2013, p. 3A.

Myung-Ok Lee, Marie. "Why I Donated My Stool." *New York Times,* July 7, 2013, p. 9.

Oaklander, Mandy, and Alice Park. "Medical Momentum: Scientists Make Major Moves in Tackling Five Challenging Diseaes." *Time,* October 27, 2014, p. 12.

O'Neal, Christopher M. Ph.D. and Raf Rizk, M.D. *Clostridium difficile: A Patient's Guide.* Inner Workings Press, 2011.

Perrone, Matthew. "FDA Eyes Unusual Medical Procedure." *Tuscaloosa* (AL) *News*, June 27, 2014, pp.1, 7A.

Sagon, Candy. "Five Medical Breakthroughs That Could Save Your Life." *AARP Magazine*, October-November 2014, pp. 23-24.

Szabo, Liz. "Gearing Up to Battle 'Nightmare Bacteria.'" USA Today, March 5, 2014, 6B.

Tucker, Miriam E. "Fecal Transfer Cures Relapsing C. diff Infection." *Internal Medicine News*, January 1, 2009, p. 24.

Made in the USA
Las Vegas, NV
06 May 2022

48527534R00098